Traoré Mahamadou

Epidemiological profile of malaria

Traoré Mahamadou

Epidemiological profile of malaria

Mékin-Sikoro community health center in Commune I of the Bamako district, 2021

ScienciaScripts

Imprint

Any brand names and product names mentioned in this book are subject to trademark, brand or patent protection and are trademarks or registered trademarks of their respective holders. The use of brand names, product names, common names, trade names, product descriptions etc. even without a particular marking in this work is in no way to be construed to mean that such names may be regarded as unrestricted in respect of trademark and brand protection legislation and could thus be used by anyone.

Cover image: www.ingimage.com

This book is a translation from the original published under ISBN 978-620-6-70082-1.

Publisher:
Sciencia Scripts
is a trademark of
Dodo Books Indian Ocean Ltd. and OmniScriptum S.R.L publishing group

120 High Road, East Finchley, London, N2 9ED, United Kingdom
Str. Armeneasca 28/1, office 1, Chisinau MD-2012, Republic of Moldova, Europe
Printed at: see last page
ISBN: 978-620-7-63009-7

Contents

DEDICACES

In the name of Allah The All-Clement The Most Merciful Praise be to Allah, who has given me the chance to see this day in good health.

I dedicate this thesis to : Allah Soubhana Wa t'Allah, from whom I have drawn all the energy, inspiration and above all the necessary spiritual foundation. It is from you that we come and it is to you that we implore assistance, without you I would not be here today, I dedicate this work to you and ask you to grant me your grace throughout my career. Guide me to the right path. **Peace and greetings on the prophet Mohammed, his noble family and companions.**

- **To my father: Kassoum Traore**

Dear father; your human qualities, your perseverance and your perfectionism make you an example of a father to me. Your rigorous education of your children, your support, your encouragement and the sacrifices you made for me have made me what I am today. I couldn't have overcome the stress of those long years of study without your advice and your prayers. No words today can express my gratitude and my deep love for you. May God give you long life and good health.

- **To my mother: Koule Traore**

Words fail me, my dear mother, to express the depth of my feelings for you. Your sacrifices, your dedication, your fighting spirit, your concern for my education and the success of your children make you an exemplary mother. This work is also the crown of your efforts and sacrifices as a mother who listens to us. I love you and will always love you. This work is also yours; may the Almighty preserve you from evil, fill you with health and give you a long life, so that we may rejoice in the fruit of this work.

- **To my brothers and sisters TRAORE**

To my other brothers and sisters Our parents sacrificed so that we could have a good education and a better future. It's time for us to try and repay them for all their hard work. This work should be an example to you, and I urge you to do better than I did; all you need is a bit of willpower and love for a job well done, and rest assured you have mine, because united for better or worse we are doomed to work hand in hand to raise high the torch of the TRAORE family. This work is the fruit of our brotherhood. May God make us grateful and courageous children. May our fraternal ties grow even closer!

To my grandmothers

Yaye Soucko, Hawa Gakou, Fatoumata Dia dit Neh

You have always ële there for us and have done so from my childhood right up to the present day and this work is also the fruit of your limitless guidance. Thanks to your advice we have learned to cultivate excellence and be maximalists.

May God bënisse you and give you a long life of santë!

- **In memory of my brother, friend and namesake Mahamadou Traore**

I would so much have liked you to be with me on this occasion but fate decided otherwise. You may no longer be with me physically but you will always remain in my heart. You were an example to us of courage, perseverance and honesty in getting the job done. I can never thank you for the efforts you made to accompany me at the difficult start of my pharmacy studies. You have left me with a great void.

I will carry you forever in my heart and I will pray ALLAH every day for the eternal rest of your soul. Dors en paix que le tout puissant vous accueille dans son paradis. Amen !!!

ACKNOWLEDGEMENTS

I would also like to thank my very dear parents for their inestimable love, trust, support and sacrifices.

I would like to express my sincere thanks to :

- **My Director, Pr Mahamadou Soumaiia Sissoko,** for agreeing to supervise me, for his advice and, above all, for his understanding.

I would also like to thank **Dr Yssouf Kone**, Technical Director of the Mekin-Sikoro Community Health Centre (DTC), for honouring me by agreeing to supervise me in his department. I would like to express my respectful gratitude to him for his availability and assistance, as well as to all the staff at the centre for their help, support and encouragement. I would also like to thank the members of the jury for taking the time to read my work.

- **To Professors Sory Ibrahima Diawara** and **Amadou Birama Niangaly**

You've always responded enthusiastically when I've needed you. I would like to take this opportunity to thank you for all your efforts on my behalf.

- **To the faculty and staff of the Faculty of Pharmacy (F.A.P.H)** For your teaching and scientific education. In addition to knowledge, you taught us know-how and interpersonal skills. We are very proud to have ëlë one of your students. Please accept our sincere gratitude.

- **To the staff of ASACOMSI :**

Thank you for your cooperation and support

Special mention to the laboratory staff

Mme Sangare Aoua Soumare ; Mr Abdoulaye Traore ; Mme Konate Assetou Guindo, Mme Coulibaly Awa Togo and all the laboratory trainees for their advice and frank collaboration.

- **DI-DRUGSTORE Pharmacy :**

Personally to the promoter of DI-DRUGSTORE Pharmacy

- **Dr Marie Germaine Constance Samake (Tanti)**

I would like to thank you sincerely for your cooperation in the preparation of this work. Please accept the expression of my deepest gratitude.

For the warm welcome she has given me in her department from the start of my introductory course in pharmacy to the present day.

Please accept my sincere thanks !!!!

The staff of the dispensary: Mme Samakë Aissata Sogore, Boukary Douyon, Constance N'Diaye, Ousmane Sanogo, Gangaly Sidibë, Amadou Diakite, Yacouba Diakite, Baba Traore, Amadou Diallo, Soumaila Sagara and Mme Toloba Sah Yanogue.

Thank you for your collaboration over the many years we have spent together.

To Dr Modibo Diakite, Dr Amadou Mouhamed Kane, Dr Amadou Bore, Dr Abdouramane Traore, Dr Fousseyni Kane, Dr Boisse Traore, Dr Balla Moussa Konte, Dr Seydou Traore

Thank you for your generous support, this work is the fruit of your many forms of support and your human qualities,

- **To all my comrades and friends**

- I- In particular to the members of the dynamic group (GD Family) of **P14 (Samuel, Amadou Timbely dit Major, Mise, Mariam dite MC, Naba, Mina, Mai, N'Faly, Aziz and Awa Thiero)**

- I- **From the fourteenth class of the Numerus Clausus (Promotion Pr Feu Drissa Diallo),** for your courtesy, sense of humour and good manners;

- I- **The opportunity** for your sympathy ;
- I- **From childhood** for your sense of good manners; I will refrain from quoting you at the risk of unintentionally omitting any name. I will always remember you as good friends with whom I spent the most memorable moments of my life. Courage and good luck in your professional life.
- **To all the students of the FAPH** The memory of the time spent with you will always be engraved in my mind. May God grant you success and long life. Thank you all.

We would like to express our deepest gratitude to all those who have contributed to the preparation of this work, whether directly or indirectly, and whose names are not mentioned.

1 INTRODUCTION

Malaria is a febrile, cholysing erythrocytopathy caused by the presence and multiplication in the erythrocytes of a hematozoan of the genus *Plasmodium*, transmitted to humans by the infecting bite of the female mosquito of the genus *Anopheles*.

Today, malaria remains a major public health problem worldwide, especially in sub-Saharan Africa [1]. Five (05) plasmodial species have been found in humans to date. These include : *Plasmodium falciparum, Plasmodium vivax, Plasmodium malariae,* the *Plasmodium ovale* complex, *Plasmodium knowlesi.* Of these, *Plasmodium falciparum* is the most common and widespread in sub-Saharan Africa, particularly in Mali, accounting for 85-90% of malaria infections, compared with 10-14% for *P. malariae* and 1% for *P. ovale* [2]. Malaria is the world's leading parasitic endemic.

In its annual report for 2022, the WHO put the number of malaria cases at 247 million, including 619,000 deaths. The African region continues to bear the heaviest burden of malaria, with 234 million cases and 593,000 deaths in 2021, and almost 80% of all malaria deaths in the region were in children under the age of 5. Four African countries account for almost half of all malaria cases worldwide: Nigeria (26.6%), the Democratic Republic of Congo (12.3%), Uganda (5.1%) and Mozambique (4.1%). Burkina Faso accounts for 3.3%, Mali 3.1% and Ghana 2.2% [3].

In Mali, malaria is the main reason for consultations in health establishments, accounting for 37.5% of all consultations. According to the local health information system, in 2021, 3,147,804 confirmed cases of malaria were recorded, including 1,025,004 serious cases, and unfortunately 1,301 deaths [4].

Its national prevalence is 19% in children under 5 [5]. It accounts for 32% of all pathologies and 22% of all deaths.

Several strategies recommended by the WHO have been adopted by Mali's National Malaria Control Programme (PNLP) to reduce the burden of malaria. These are essentially curative and preventive strategies that are helping to reduce the burden of malaria in many regions [6] :

- Prevention through the use of long-lasting insecticidal nets (LLINs) ;
Intra-domiciliary spraying with insecticides (IDP);
- Intermittent preventive treatment in pregnant women (IPT) ;
- Chemoprevention of seasonal malaria (CPS) in children and adolescents
tlierape'utic combinations based on artemisinin (CTA).

However, malaria remains one of the leading causes of child mortality, killing one child every two minutes worldwide [7].

Malaria indicators enable rigorous monitoring of the disease to assess the effectiveness of the various prevention and treatment measures. Numerous cross-sectional studies have been conducted on malaria indicators in Mali. However, this type of study, although instructive, does not provide information on malaria management at health facility level.

We therefore undertook this study to evaluate the management of malaria at the Mekin-Sikoro CSCOM.

OBJECTIVES :

1.1 General objective :

To evaluate the management of malaria in the population of Мёкт-Sikoro in 2021.

1.2 Specific objectives :

- Dëterminer la frequence du paludisme au CSCOM de Mëкт-Sikoro en 2021 ;
- Identifying the clinical and biological profile of malaria in the CSCOM of Mëкт-Sikoro in 2021;
- Dëcrire le schëma tlérapeutique utilisë au CSCOM de Mëкт-Sikoro en 2021 ;
- Dëterminer la frequence d'utilisation des mesures de prevention du paludisme par les patients/ accompagnants au CSCOM de Mëкт-Sikoro en 2021 ;
- Dë determine patients'/carers' knowledge of how malaria is transmitted.

2 General information

2.1 Etymology :

Malaria, from the Latin "palus" (swamp), also appelë malaria, from the Italian "mal'aria" (bad air) is a parasitosis transmitted by the bite of a mosquito, *dAnopheles* which breeds in wetlands. The parasites responsible are protists belonging to the *Plasmodium* genus. It is the most common vector-borne infectious disease in the hot tropical regions of Africa, Latin America and Asia. In these regions, climatic and environmental conditions are conducive to the development of mosquitoes, particularly female anopheles, the sole vector of *Plasmodium*. Plasmodium is primarily a human disease. However, *Plasmodium* also infects birds, reptiles, monkeys, chimpanzees and rodents (warm-blooded animals) **[8]**.

2.2 Historical background:

Malaria is probably one of the oldest known human diseases, with clinical manifestations dating back to ancient times. The Italian terms Mal' aria, "bad air", and Latin paludis, "marsh", were written by Hippocrates (460-377 BC), among others, who also established a relevant relationship between the date and the place where the patients lived when they died **[9]**.

The presence of *P falciparum* has been demonstrated in Egyptian mummies dating back 3000 years BC (Chastel, 2004). From the fourth century onwards, the Chinese used the Qinghaosu tree or Artemisia annua for its fëbrifugal properties. In 1620, Don Francisco Lopez, the next Jë father, recognised the curative properties of cinchona bark powder and distinguished between fevers that reacted favourably and those that did not. The "Jësuites powder" was a huge success, as malaria ëик was widespread in Europe at the time. As early as 1717, Lancisi incriminated mosquitoes, claiming that "malaria is due to a marsh poison transmitted by mosquitoes that inoculate the blood with bad humours".

In 1820, Pelletier and Caventou isolated two active cinchona alkaloids, quinine and cinchonine. In 1880 Alphonse Laveran, a French military doctor, observed intrarerythrocytic cellular elements in Algeria that did not belong to any hëmatological lig^e; the malaria parasite was discovered. The distinction between the species *Plasmodium malariae, Plasmodium vivax* and *Plasmodium falciparum* was made between 1885 and 1890 by Golgi, Marchiafava, Grassi and Felleti in Italy.

In 1897, the British physician Sir Ronald Ross of l'aттёe India proved the role of mosquitoes in the transmission of avian malaria **[10]**, and Giovanni-Batista Grassi, in 1898 in Italy, demonstrated that the anophële is the vector of human malaria. In 1900, Schaudinn described and named the stages in the *Plasmodium* cycle. In 1922, Stephens described *Plasmodium ovale*. Now that the parasite had been discovered, its mode of transmission had to be determined. The division phase in the liver was not identified until much later, in 1948, by Short and Garnham. They thus made it possible to computerise knowledge of the parasite's cycle and to explain the relapses of the disease observed in certain cases.

The last stage of the life cycle, the presence of dormant stages in the liver, was conclusively demonstrated in 1982 by Wojciech Krotoski **[11]**.

The Second World War prevented access to the cinchona plantations in Indonesia, paving the way for the development and use of the first synthetic antimalarials (4-aminoquinolines). Control of the vector became possible thanks to the discovery of insecticides with a remanent action, which enabled the disease to be eradicated in parts of Europe still affected, and in certain islands. Resistance was to appear rapidly, ruining malaria eradication experiments.

2.3 Epidemiology :
2.3.1 Epidemiological background :
They assess the frequency and distribution of malaria within a given population, making it possible to define different levels of transmission and endemicity, and thus to adapt malaria control strategies to the biotope under consideration.

Malaria affects around a hundred countries around the world, particularly the poor tropical areas of Africa, Asia and Latin America. The epidemiology of malaria can vary considerably even within a relatively small geographical area. It is influenced by factors relating to the human host, the vector, the parasite and environmental factors. These are essentially genetic factors influencing the host's susceptibility to plasmodial infections, the vectorial capacities of anopheles and their resistance to insecticides, the parasites' ability to resist antimalarial drugs and the evasion of the host's immune system. Environmental factors, particularly climate, rainfall and relief, are thought to influence vector survival. Abrupt changes in environmental factors are at the root of malaria epidemics.

The ëpidëmiology of malaria involves the study of four (4) elements whose simultaneous reunion is essential for the development of the disease:
- The presence of men carrying *Plasmodium* gametocytes in their peripheral blood,
- The existence of a population of anophëles vectors,
- The presence of men receptive to *Plasmodium,*
- Favourable ecological conditions

2.3.2 Geographical distribution :
Malaria is widespread throughout the intertropical world, with the three main areas of high transmission being sub-Saharan Africa, South-East Asia and South America. There are currently 87 countries in which malaria is endemic, or transmission is continuous. Of the countries affected by malaria, 46 reported fewer than 10,000 cases of malaria in 2019, compared with 26 countries in 2000. By the end of 2020, 24 countries had reported an interruption of malaria transmission for at least three years, 11 of which have been certified malaria-free by the WHO [12].

Europe :

Malaria has been eradicated in Europe, including the Azores, the Canary Islands, Cyprus, Eastern Europe and the European part of Turkey. In 2011, *P. vivax* reappeared in Greece (autochthonous cases). It should be noted that cases of airport malaria are sometimes described in connection with the importation of infested mosquitoes in the luggage or cabins of aircraft from endemic areas.

America :

In the Americas, there has been increased transmission in Brazil, Nicaragua and especially Venezuela, where the situation is clearly deteriorating. There is a high proportion of *P. vivax* infection (in French Guiana: *P. falciparum*: 45%, *P. vivax*: 55%) [13].

Asia :

The whole of South-East Asia (Myanmar, South China, Thailand, Vietnam, Cambodia, Laos, Malaysia, Indonesia and the Philippines) is endemic to malaria caused by : *Plasmodium falciparum, Plasmodium vivax*, and *Plasmodium knowlesi*. The other regions and the Indian peninsula are

P. vivax and *P. falciparum* but are not affected by the phënomëne of multidrug resistance. Transmission in Asia takes the form of outbreaks: disseminated in rural areas in wooded hilly zones. All major Asian cities are free of the disease (except Indian cities).

Oceania :

Transmission is heterogeneous. Some areas, such as New Gurnee, the Solomon Islands and Vanuatu, are free of the disease, while others, such as French Polynesia, New Caledonia, Wallis and Futuna, Fiji, Hawaii, Australia and New Zealand, are completely free **[13]**.

Near and Middle East :

Plasmodium falciparum occurs on the west coast of the Arabian Peninsula and in Yemen. All cities are free of the disease, as are Bahrain, Is^l, Jordan, Lebanon, Kuwait and Qatar. The risk is low in other states such as Syria, south-east Turkey, the United Arab Emirates and Oman **[13]**.

Africa:

Malaria exists to a small extent in North Africa, where the species *P vivax* and *P malariae* are found. It is widespread throughout intertropical Africa, where *P falciparum*, *P. ovale* and, to a lesser extent, *P. malariae* coexist. In certain areas of East Africa, *P vivax is* also found. Transmission is intense in Madagascar, where all four species co-exist. Generally speaking, areas of high endemicity in Africa start in the Sahara sub-region and extend into the equatorial zone.

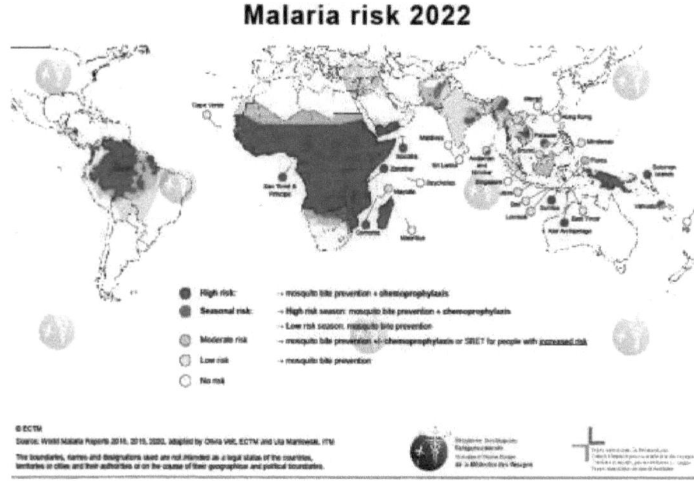

Figure 1: Geographical distribution of malaria in the world

Available at: https://www.wanda.be/fr/a-z-index/malaria-carte-du-monde

In Mali, there are 5 epidemiological types of malaria transmission [15].

> A Sudanese-Guianese zone with seasonal transmission lasting 6 months. Malaria is holo-endëmic with a Plasmodic Index (PI) of around 85% from June to November. Premunition is acquired at around 5 years of age.

> A short seasonal transmission zone of 3 to 4 months. This corresponds to the northern Sudanian zone and the Sahel. Malaria is hyper-endëmic here, with a Plasmodium index varying between 50 and 75%. Premunition is reached around the age of 9, and neuromalaria is one of the most frequent complications between the ages of 1 and 9.

> The bi- or multi-modal transmission zones include the inland delta of the River Niger and the dam zones: Sëlinguë, Manantali and Markala. Malaria is endemic in these areas, with a prevalence rate of less than 40%. The prevalence of malaria anaemia is very high in the under-9 age group.

> Areas that are not conducive to malaria: urban areas (Bamako, Mopti, etc.). Malaria in these areas is hypo-endëmic, with a PI of less than 10%. Adults in Bamako are also at risk of severe malaria.

> An area of sporadic or even epidemic transmission corresponding to the northern regions and certain localities in the Koulikoro and Kayes regions (Nara, Nioro, Diëma, Yëlimanë, Kayes). The lP is below 5%. All age groups are at risk of severe malaria. A parйcиHёre precaution must be taken whenever these populations migrate to the south of the country; even adults in this area are at risk of severe and complicated malaria.

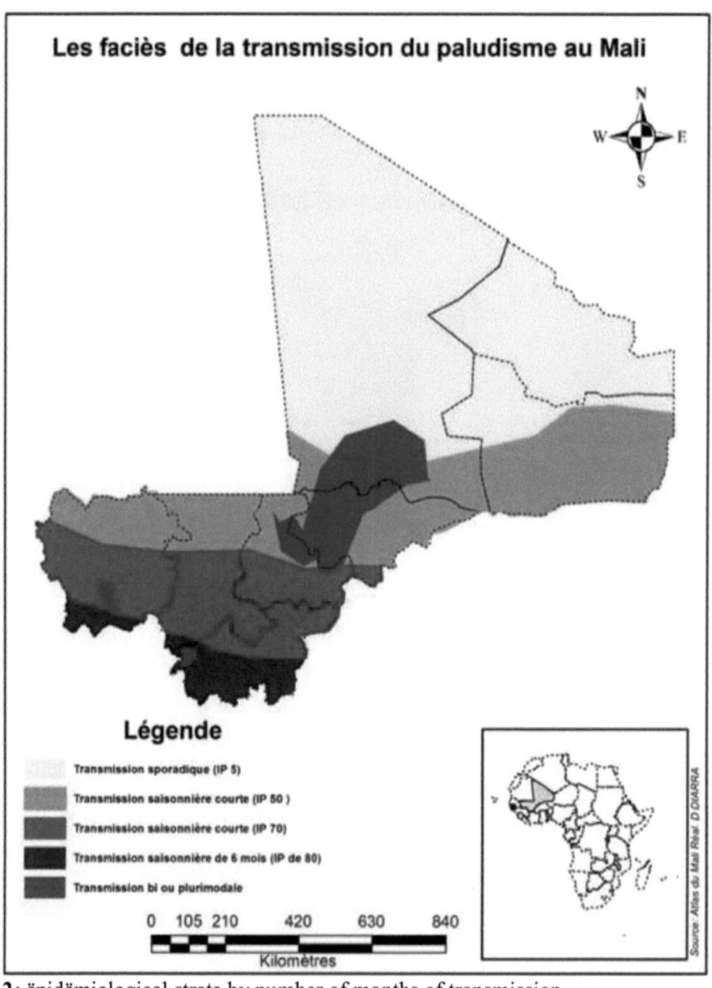

Figure 2: ëpidëmiological strata by number of months of transmission.

2.3.3 Pathogens :

Taxonomic classification of *Plasmodium* :

Subrange: *Protozoa*

Phylum : *Apicomplexa*

Class: *sporozoa*

Subclass: *Coccidia*

Superclass: *Eucoccidia*

Order: *Eucocciddida*

Suborder: *Haemosporina*

Family: *Plasmodiidae*

Genus: *Plasmodium*

Species: *P. falciparum, P. vivax, P. ovale* (subspecies *P ovale Walkeri, P. ovale curtisi), P. malariae, P. knowlesi.*

Malaria is caused by parasites of the genus *Plasmodium* and transmitted by female mosquitoes belonging to the genus *Anopheles*. *Plasmodiums* are protozoa belonging to the phylum Sporozoa, the order *Haemosporidae*, the class *Haemosporidae* and the family *Plasmodidae*. Three players are needed for malaria to develop: the pathogen (the parasite), the vector (the mosquito) and the host (man). In addition to these 3 players, there are the favourable ecological conditions.

There are many species of *Plasmodium* (over 140), affecting various animal species, but the most frequently encountered in human pathology are : *P. falciparum, P. vivax, P. ovale curtisi (Poc), P. ovale wallikeri (Pow), P. malariae, P. knowlesi.* The last two species are parasites usually described in Asian monkeys but which have recently been discovered in humans [7]. The different species of *Plasmodium* differ according to biological and clinical criteria, geographical distribution and their ability to develop resistance to antimalarial drugs. *P. falciparum* is the species most commonly found in Africa, is responsible for potentially fatal clinical forms, especially in vulnerable groups, and is the species most implicated in resistance to antimalarial drugs [16].

The five (5) plasmodial species infected with humans are [17]: *Plasmodium falciparum, Plasmodium vivax, Plasmodium ovale, Plasmodium malariae and Plasmodium knowlesi.*

Plasmodium falciparum: This is responsible for malignant third fever [18]. This is the most dreaded species and the most widespread. It is responsible for almost all malaria cases, and is the most widespread and formidable plasmodial species in the world, especially in tropical and subtropical areas. It accounts for 85-90% of the parasite formula in Mali. It is the most prevalent malaria parasite in sub-Saharan Africa. It was responsible for 99% of malaria cases estimated in 2016. Transmission is annual in equatorial regions, with seasonal upsurges, while in subtropical regions it occurs only during hot, humid periods.

P. falciparum is responsible for potentially fatal clinical forms, in particular neuromalaria. The incubation period is 7-12 days [19].

Plasmodium vivax [20] is the second most common species of human malaria parasite, affecting an estimated 75 million people each year. However, it is very rare in West and Central Africa, due to the high prevalence of the Duffy-negative phenotype (mostly West

Africans), who do not possess the membrane receptor necessary for *P. vivax* infection. Recently, cases of *P. vivax* infection have been described in Africa **[21]**. **The** clinical manifestations associated with *P. vivax* are classically considered benign, but sometimes with relapses. The incubation period is 11 to 13 days, often with late relapses **[19]**.

Plasmodium malariae Occurs much more sporadically in Africa, accounting for 10 to 14%, and is the agent of quarantine fever. It is mainly responsible for very late relapses (up to 20 years after returning from the endemic zone).

The pathophysiological mechanisms of these late forms are not fully elucidated, although some suggest the presence of latent merozoites in the lymphatic tract. The clinical manifestations of the infection are benign, but can sometimes lead to renal complications. The incubation period can range from 15 to 21 days.

Discovered in 1880 by the Frenchman Alphonse Laveran, it differs from the other three human plasmodia in that it develops slowly, due to a less pronounced schizogony.

prolific. The asexual cycle lasts 72 hours instead of 48 hours in the other three species;

This is why the malaria-like illness attributed to it is known as quarte fever.

All stages (trophozoites, schizonts, gametocytes) are found in peripheral blood. Under the light microscope, on a thin or thick Giemsa-stained smear, the young trophozoites are in rings and at this stage do not differ from the corresponding forms of *P. vivax*, but the parasites do not take long to elongate and spread out in transverse bands, characteristic of this species. A thick, dark blue ring can be seen. The hemozoin pigment (yellowish) appears very early and is more visible than in other parasites. Gametocytes resemble those of *P. vivax* but are smaller and more pigmented. Parasitic erythrocytes retain their usual shape (thin smear). *P. malariae* can survive for a very long time in peripheral blood (10 years or more) at a low level of parasitemia, occasionally producing a recrudescence of clinical symptoms **[22]**.

Plasmodium ovale: accounts for less than 1%. It is responsible for benign third stage fever. It is found mainly in regions where *P vivax* is absent or rare (black Africa). This species does not kill but causes relapses several years (2 to 5 years) after sporozoal inoculation **[23]**.

Plasmodium knwolesi: responsible for monkey malaria, which has recently been shown to be transmitted to humans.

P. cynomolgi infects macaque monkeys like *P. knowlesi,* and is mainly found in South-East Asia.

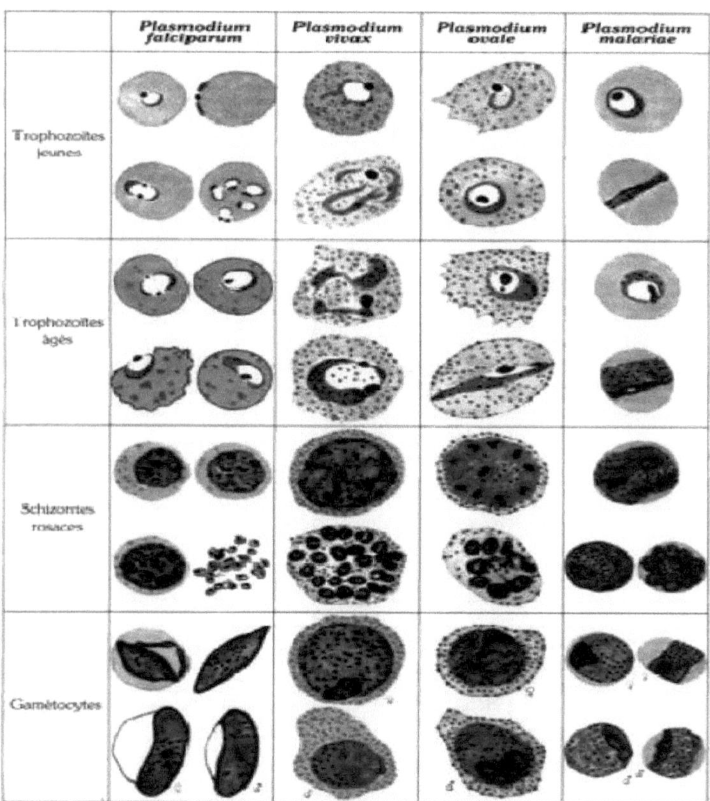

Figure 3: *Plasmodium* at various stages. Aspects on thin smear.
<u>Source:</u> Anne-Marie Deluol, H. Levillayer, Jean-Louis Poirot.

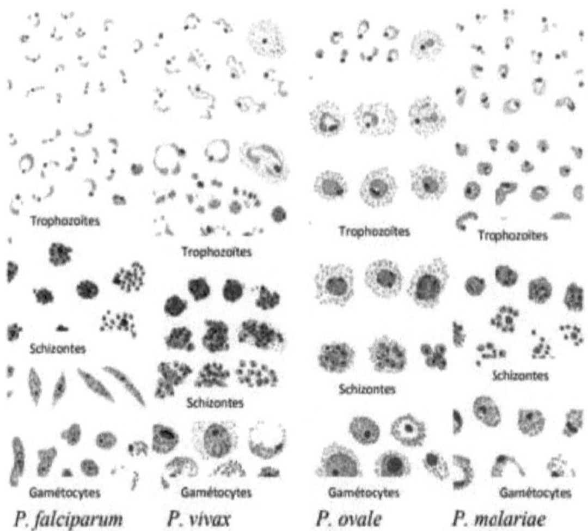

Figure 4: *Plasmodium* at various stages. Aspects on ëpais smears.

<u>Source</u>: F. Castelli, G. Carosi

2.3.4 Vectors :

The malaria vector is a *culicidea* mosquito of the genus *Anopheles*. There are many vector species, and they are all the more formidable because they are very sensitive to humans (anthropophilic species). They feed and rest in houses (endophilic or domiciliary species). Only the hematophagous female is responsible for transmission.

To date, 484 species have been identified, but only around sixty of these are vectors of malaria in humans. The main vector involved is anopheles gambiae on the African continent, where it cohabits with A. *funestus* and A. *arabiensis* [24].

In Mali, members of the *Anopheles gambiae s.l and Anopheles funestus* complex generally transmit malaria between 18 and 6 o'clock in the morning [25].

The nature of the soil, the rainfall pattern, the temperature and therefore the altitude, the natural vegetation or agriculture, make water nests more or less suitable for the development of vector species. Some species have thus been able to adapt to particular environments, such as the urban environment. The development and longevity of anopheles depend on temperature, with an optimum between 20 and 30°C for a life span of around 30 days [26].

2.3.5 Transmission of malaria

All malaria vector species bite between dusk and dawn. The intensity of transmission depends on factors Hё3 to the parasite, the vector, the host (man) and the environment. *Anopheles* lay their eggs in water. These eggs hatch into larvae and then become adult mosquitoes. Female mosquitoes look for a blood meal to feed their eggs. Each species has its own prëfèrences regarding its aquatic habitat; some, for example, preëfèrent small shallow freshwater quant^s, such as puddles and animal hoof prints, which are found in abundance during the rainy season in tropical countries. Transmission is most intense where mosquito species are long-lived (allowing the parasite to complete its development cycle inside the mosquito) and where they tend to bite humans rather than animals. The long lifespan and high preëfèrence to humans of African vector species are among the reasons why around 90% of malaria cases worldwide occur in Africa [27].

Transmission also depends on climatic conditions that can influence mosquito abundance and survival; for example, rainfall patterns, tempĕrature and humidity. In many places, transmission is seasonal with a peak occurring during or just after the rainy season. Malaria outbreaks can occur when climate and other conditions suddenly favour transmission in areas where populations have little or no immunity. Malaria epidemics can also occur when people with low immunity move to areas of intense transmission.

2.3.6 The evolutionary cycle of *Plasmodium* :

The cycle unfolds successively in the male (asexual phase in the intermediary host) and in the anophyte (sexual phase in the definitive host) [28].

In humans

The cycle is divided into two phases:

•   The hĕpatic or prererythrocytic or exorerythrocytic phase corresponds to the incubation phase, clinically asymptomatic;

•   The blood or ërythrocytic phase, which corresponds to the clinical phase of the disease.

The hepatic phase: The sporozoites inoculated by the female anopheles during its blood meal remain in the skin, lymph and blood for a maximum of thirty minutes. Many are dĕtruit by macrophages, but some manage to reach hĕpatocytes [28]. They transform into pre-erythrocytic schizonts or "blue bodies" (multinucleate forms) which, after a few days of maturation, burst open and release thousands of mĕrozoites into the blood (10,000 to 30,000 depending on the species).

In the blood, each mĕrozoite pĕnĕtreats into the red blood cell and becomes a trophozoite which grows, forming a schizont and then a rosette body. This bursts open, releasing mĕrozoites which infest new red blood cells. They transform again into trophozoites and then into rosette bodies which burst, infecting other red blood cells, and so on. The synchronous bursting of the rosette bodies, every 48 or 72 hours depending on the species, corresponds to febrile acces. After several endo-erythrocytic cycles of this type, some trophozoites transform into female and male gametocytes ingested by the female anopheles [29].

In *P. vivax* and *P. ovale* infections, delayed hepatic schizogony (hypnozoites) may lead to the release of merozoites into the blood several months after the mosquito bite, thus explaining the late relapses observed with these two species [28].

The erythrocyte phase: This part of the cycle corresponds to the clinical phase.

Merozoites released during the hepatic phase penetrate the red blood cells. The penetration of the merozoite into the erythrocyte and its maturation into a trophozoite and then a schizont is species-dependent and leads to the destruction of the host red blood cell and the release of 8 to 32 new merozoites [28]. These merozoites penetrate new red blood cells and begin a new replication cycle.

After a certain number of erythrocytic cycles, gametocytogenesis occurs. Gametocytogenesis is a process that leads some parasites to stop the cell cycle and initiate a phase of cellular differentiation into sexual forms.

The mechanisms by which the merozoite differentiates into a gametocyte are poorly understood. The main marker of commitment to the gametocytic pathway is the development of a vacuole and microtubules responsible for the elongation and symmetry of the microorganism [30].

The number of gametocytes is usually much lower than in asexual stages, in the order of 1 to

3 gametocytes per 100 trophozoites **[31]**.

In female anopheles

In the female anopheles, which is the only matophagous mosquito, a sex cycle or sporogony takes place. The mosquito sucks blood containing gametocytes from humans. The male gametocyte will emit 6 to 8 flagellate gametes which will fecundate female gametes to give rise to a reproductive unit called an ookinete. This mobile egg will pass through the gastric wall of the anopheles and encyst on the outside, forming an oocyst. Inside the oocyst, the nuclei divide, producing hundreds or thousands of sporozoites that reach the mosquito's salivary glands. The mosquito is then infesting and can transmit malaria to a receptive individual when bitten. The average duration of the sporogonic cycle is fifteen days, but can vary from ten to forty days depending on temperature, humidity and the anopheline and plasmodial species involved.

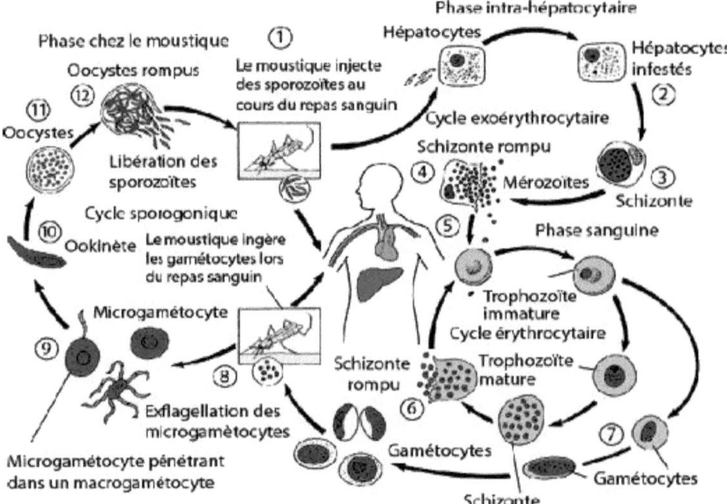

Figure 5: *Plasmodium* life cycle
<u>**Source:**</u> **https://www.merckmanuals.com/fr-ca [32]** ANOFEL 2014

2.3.7 Pathophysiology of malaria :

The pathophysiology of malaria is still imperfectly understood, but the repercussions of malaria infection on certain organs have been well described:

The blood

The ërythrocytic schizogony phase leads to hëmolysis responsible for severe anemia, which progressively sets in in pregnant women and young children. The haemoglobin destroyed by haemolysis is converted into bilirubin in the liver. As bilirubin is produced in excës, it is eliminated by the liver, causing renal overload and resulting in haemoglobinuria.

On the other hand, the parasite present in the hematite uses the lierne and causes it to precipitate in the form of pigment granules called hemozoin, the release of which when the erythrocyte bursts is partly responsible for the fiëvre. The pigment, accumulated in the cytoplasm of the schizont, is released into the plasma when the merozoites are released. It is then phagocytosed by monocyte-macrophages and neutrophil polynuclears (melaniferous leukocytes).

Platelets are sequestered by mechanisms that are as yet unclear, and are probably immunological. The consequence is thrombocytopenia, a biological disturbance frequently and early observed during a malaria attack.

- **Spleen**

The spleen becomes enlarged in the case of infections, anaemia and cancer in some individuals who live in an area where it becomes soft and congestive. This increase in volume is caused by hypertrophy of the white pulp (lymphocytes, reticular cells, macrophages). Pigment phagocyted by monocyte-macrophages and neutrophil polynuclears accumulates in the spleen, giving it a dark red, sometimes brown, colour. This erythrophagocytosis is accelerated by two phenomena: the activation of macrophages and the binding of immunoglobulins to the wall of erythrocytes, whether infected or not. It is easy to rupture because of the increased fragility of the capsule.

Histologically, in evolving visceral malaria, the spleen is huge, fibro-congestive and dark on section, with lymphoid and histiocytic hyperplasia, but parasites are rare.

Splenomegaly is a sign that accompanies the development of parasitemia. It forms the basis of an epidemiometric observation: the splenic index. This gives an account of the frequency of enlarged spleens in a population and is a measure of malaria endemia in a given area.

Kidneys

The formation of antigen-antibody complexes and their deëpôt in the basement membrane causes kidney overload and a reduction in the depuration capacity of this organ, which is already abnormally strained in the event of haemolysis. Thrombosis of the arterioles of the renal glomeruli, anoxia of the surrounding tubular cells and signs of glomerulonephritis are frequently observed. Local degeneration is possible, leading to nephrosis (a frequent complication in *P. malariae*). The main danger of hemoglobinuric bilious fever is renal blockage due to massive destruction of red blood cells.

- **The central nervous system**

The deep schizogony of *P. falciparum* is the cause of formidable complications, including cerebral malaria. This consists of capillary thrombosis responsible for vascular and haemorrhagic lesions, causing degenerative alterations to nerve cells, surrounded by cellular infiltrates. There are several theories to explain these phenomena:

• The presence of mechanical obstacles in the micro-capillary and venous circulation results in reduced deformability of the parasitic erythrocytes and the formation of "rosettes" consisting of a parasitic red blood cell to which normal erythrocytes adhere by an unclear mechanism (antigens and immunoglobulins exposed on its surface are thought to play a role). These phenomena cause a reduction in circulatory flow and a reversible metabolic coma [33].

• The immunological adhesion of parasitic globules to the postcapillary vascular endothelium causes major circulatory slowdowns. This adhesion is thought to depend on certain parasite cell surface proteins visible under the electron microscope (protuberances or "knobs"), CD4+ T lymphocytes, certain interleukins, in particular TNF, and endothelial receptors of the ICAM-1 type.

• Symptoms will include hemiplegia or convulsions (motor areas), thermoregulatory disorders with hyperpyrexia (hypothalamus), and progressive alteration of consciousness if the whole brain is involved.

The placenta

Placental villi are surrounded by large sinuses where maternal blood circulates slowly. The spaces between the villi are an excellent refuge for red blood cells parasitised by *P. falciparum*. The accumulation of parasitic blood cells, attached to each other and destroyed on the spot, creates a call for macrophages. This engorgement can cause a blockage of the interstitial spaces and placental thrombosis. The reduction in freto-maternal exchanges is one of the reasons why chemoprophylaxis is recommended for pregnant women: its aim is to reduce the number of parasites in circulation.

Anemia results from the bursting of parasitic red blood cells. Hepatomegaly and splenomegaly are due to hyperactivity of the monocyte-macrophage system responsible for clearing malarial pigment and erythrocyte debris [34].

2.3.8 Clinical manifestations of malaria

Acces malustre de primo-invasion a *P. falciparum* [35] :

This is the clinical form most often seen in mainland France, as it affects new, non-immune individuals, such as travellers. In endemic areas, it is seen in young children.

-       Incubation: This corresponds to the duration of the hepatocytic phase (7 to 12 days for *P. falciparum)* and is completely asymptomatic.

-       Invasion: This is marked by the appearance of a sudden, continuous fever, often accompanied by general malaise with myalgia, headache and sometimes digestive problems (anorexia, abdominal pain, nausea, vomiting and sometimes even diarrhoea). This is known as "febrile gastric embarrassment".

At this stage, the clinical examination is often normal, and the liver and spleen are not palpable. Later, the liver may increase in size and become slightly painful, the spleen becomes palpable after a few days, urine is rare, dark and may contain protein. A patch of herpes labialis is sometimes seen. The clinical picture is therefore totally non-specific, and the major risk is of "missing the diagnosis" if there is no record of a trip to an endemic area. However, the patient can, at any time and in the space of a few hours, progress from a "simple attack" (i.e. uncomplicated) to a serious attack, which can rapidly lead to death if not treated appropriately. At the start of an episode, there is no epidemiological, clinical or biological evidence to enable a prognosis to be made or to know whether or not a patient will progress to a severe case. Consequently, the diagnosis of malaria is a medical emergency: "any fever in a patient returning from a malaria-endemic area is malaria until proven otherwise".

Malaria attack: This clinical form corresponds to the description of the classic malaria attack triad: **"chills, heat, sweats"** occurring every 2 or 3 days. In practice, it is only typically observed in *P. vivax, P. ovale and P. malariae* infestations, following an untreated primary invasion, but may occur long after the initial febrile episode [36].

Severe malaria:

P. falciparum malaria in non-immune individuals (young children in endemic areas, pregnant women, expatriates, travellers) is potentially fatal. Death, when it occurs, is secondary to the failure of one or more major functions, sometimes even if etiological treatment has proved effective. Only the rapid initiation of appropriate resuscitation can save the patient. It is therefore absolutely essential to know the severity criteria for *P falciparum* malaria, in order to identify patients who warrant emergency hospitalisation, if necessary in an Intensive Care Unit. Severe malaria can therefore take a variety of clinical forms, the most important of which is cerebral involvement. The term "cerebral malaria" is used to describe all the neurological manifestations resulting from cerebral involvement during malaria attacks: disturbances of consciousness, prostration and convulsions.

- The onset may be gradual or brutal, with pernicious attack with a gradual onset marked by the onset of irregular fever and a diffuse algic syndrome, associated with digestive disorders. The clinical examination may already reveal a neurological component, suggesting progression to severe malaria.

In clinical practice: "any patient presenting with impaired consciousness or any other sign of cerebral dysfunction on return from a malaria-endemic area should be treated as a neuromalarial case as a matter of the utmost urgency". A pernicious attack with a sudden onset results in a triad of symptoms (fever, coma, convulsions), frequently accompanied by respiratory distress. It is common in young children in endemic areas and can lead to death within a few hours.

- During the state phase, fever is usually very high and the neurological picture often associated with it is :

• **Disturbances of consciousness**: these are constant but of varying intensity, ranging from simple obnubilation to deep coma. The coma is generally calm, without neck rigidity (or very discreet), without photophobia, and accompanied by abolition of the corneal reflex.

• **Convulsions**: much more frequent in children than in adults; they may be inaugural. They may be generalized or localized, spaced out over time or, on the contrary, may represent a convulsive state. They may sometimes be paucisymptomatic (clonic lips, facial muscles, rapid eye movements, excessive salivation).

They must be distinguished from hyperthermic convulsions: to be considered, they must be repeated over time (> 2 / 24 hours) with a postcritical phase > 15 minutes.

• **Tonus disorders**: the patient is generally hypotonic. Stiffness and opisthotonos may be seen in very advanced forms and have a poor prognosis. Osteotendinous reflexes are variable, sometimes very sharp, exceptionally abolished (poor prognosis).

• **Other associated clinical signs**: neurological signs may dominate the clinical picture or be associated with other visceral manifestations. Virtually all organs may be affected, in particular the kidneys, lungs (risk of pulmonary redeme) and liver. The picture is sometimes one of multivisceral failure. Sometimes, without any obvious neurological signs, severe forms are observed, with profound anemia (in children) or acute renal failure (in adults).

- **Evolution**

If left untreated, neuromalaria is fatal in two or three days. With appropriate treatment, the mortality rate remains high (10-30%). When this is achieved, recovery is generally without sequelae, except in children (5-10% of definitive sequelae). The overall prognosis depends essentially on the speed of diagnosis.

<u>**WHO severity criteria**</u>

The WHO defined criteria for the severity of malaria in 2000. The presence of just one of these criteria, clinical or biological, combined with the presence of *P. falciparum in* the blood, leads to the diagnosis of severe malaria as shown in table 1:

Table 1: Sëvëres forms of malaria according to WHO in 2014 [37].

Consciousness disorders	**Modified Glasgow score <9 in adults and children over 5 Blantyre score <2 in small children**
Repeated convulsions	**> 2/ 24 hours (despite correction of**

	hyperthermia)
Prostration	Extreme weakness Or in children: inability to sit up for a child old enough to do so, or to drink for a child too young to sit up.
Respiratory distress	Clinical definition
Ictere	Clinical or biological (bilirubin >50 pmol/L)
Macroscopic haemoglobinuria	Dark red or black urine; haemoglobinuria or myoglobinuria on dipstick. Absence of microscopic haematuria.
Circulatory collapse	SBP<80mmHg in adults SBP<50mmHg in children
pulmonary ffideme	Radiological definition
Abnormal bleeding	
Severe anemia	Adult: Hb <7g/dl or Hte <20%. Child: Hb <5g/dl or Hte<15%.
Hypoglycemia	Blood glucose <2.2 mmol/L
Metabolic Acidosis	Ph <7.35 or bicarbonates <15mmol/L
Consciousness disorders	(Glasgow score 9)
Hyperparasitemia	>40% non-immune subject
Renal insufficiency	Creatinemia > 265 pmol/L after rehydration Or diuresis < 400 ml/24h in adults (<12mL/kg/24h in children)

National policy guidelines on the diagnosis and treatment of malaria cases in Mali's ComHCs :

The ComHCs, which are the first level of contact between the health services and the population, must be equipped with the means to diagnose malaria biologically (laboratory facilities for thick drop and smear tests, and rapid diagnostic test kits). They manage cases of uncomplicated malaria and refer patients as soon as danger signs appear. They also manage cases of malaria in the rest of the population, including pregnant women, in accordance with the standards set out in the national policy.

2.3.9 Biological diagnosis

Diagnosis of malaria consists of identifying the blood forms of the parasite. Blood samples should be taken as close as possible to the thermal peak [38].

2.3.9.1 Direct diagnosis :

This is the optical microscopic examination of blood samples taken preferably before any antimalarial treatment, at the time of febrile peaks.

- Thick drop (GE)

A World Health Organisation (WHO) reference test, it is widely used for routine diagnosis. Its sensitivity (2 parasites per mm3) is 10 to 20 times greater than that of the thin smear (20 parasites/pl detectable).

The procedure consists of taking a drop of blood from a finger prick on an object blade and immediately defibrillating it with a spiral movement using a corner of another blade not yet in use. This movement will spread the blood over an area approximately one centimetre in diameter. The sample is dried and then stained, without prior fixation, using an aqueous solution of Giemsa, which has a staining action. After staining, only the leukocytes and any parasites remain on the slide. The thick drop of blood is used to cover a larger volume of blood to make the diagnosis and avoid missing *Plasmodium.*

A negative test must be repeated within 12 to 24 hours, if clinical suspicion persists.

- Thin smear (FM): used for morphological studies of hëmatozoa and differential diagnosis between plasmodial species.

The slide is stained using the May-Grunwald-Giemsa method or with Giemsa after fixation with alcohol. The parasites, stained red (nucleus) and blue (cytoplasm), are found inside the red blood cells (no haemolysis in this technique). However, the amount of blood examined is smaller than for a thick drop, and this method may not work in cases where parasitemia is low.

Its disadvantage is that it does not detect low-density parasitemia (100 to 300 parasites/microlitre of blood). The ideal diagnostic approach would involve microscopic examination of a blood smear and a thickened drop (2007 Revision of the 1999 Consensus Conference).

The QBC (Quantitative Buffy Coat)

This is a direct immunofluorescence method. The principle involves concentrating a small quantity of blood by centrifugation in a micro hematocrit tube. Parasite red blood cells are also found at the interface between leukocytes and healthy red blood cells. The orange acridine, a specific nucleic acid intercalating agent, contained in the nuclei causes the parasite to fluoresce green or yellow-orange inside the red blood cell. It is of interest in pauciparasitic forms, for monitoring the progress of infection **[39]**.

Its main drawback is the difficulty of establishing a species diagnosis. In addition, the need for a fluorescence microscope may limit small structures in the acquisition of this device.

Detection of malaria antigens by rapid diagnostic tests (RDT)

Rapid diagnostic tests (RDTs) have facilitated access to diagnosis, reversing the paradigm of "any febrile patient is considered to have malaria" in areas where microscopy was not available **[40][41].**

Several tests of this type are on the market. They are based on the principle of immunochromatography, using strips sensitised with specific monoclonal antibodies detecting plasmodial antigens **[42]**. They are performed using a drop of blood deposited on a cassette and do not require any equipment.

-    **Detection of Ag histidine rich protein 2 (HRP2):** this *P. falciparum* species-specific glycoprotein is produced by all asexual ërythrocytic stages of the parasite,

-    **Lactate Dehydrogenase(pLDH),** an enzyme that *Plasmodium* uses in the production of energy. This enzyme can be specific to *P. falciparum, P. vivax* and can also be specific to all plasmodial species (pan-specific);

-    **Aldolase,** an enzyme used by all plasmodial species (pan-specific);

On the market, the various TDRs come in four formats:

-    Strips
-    Plastic cassettes
-    Cards
-    Mixed format, cassette-tape.

Their detection thresholds vary from 100 to 200 parasites/pl [45]. **The** major disadvantages of these tests are the persistence of the antigenemia after recovery and their mono-specificity with respect to *P. falciparum*. False positives have also been associated with cross-reactivity with rheumatoid factors [46]. False negatives are possible and are thought to be due to mutations in the gene coding for HRP2 or to the presence of antibodies [47] directed against the parasite lactate dehydrogenase (LDH).

RDTs are quick to perform and easy to read, and can be carried out by moderately trained staff. They are particularly useful in non-specialist facilities where microscopic examination is not available [48]. Their performance depends essentially on the parasitemia [49]. They are also less effective with species other than *P falciparum,* particularly *P ovale* [50]. RDTs should be considered as a complement to other diagnostic methods. Their results must be verified and, if possible, supplemented by microscopic examination. If they are positive, patients can be managed appropriately and rapidly. On the other hand, if they are negative, the diagnosis should not be ruled out [51].

Diagnosis using molecular biology

This method is based on the detection of parasite nucleic acids by polymerase chain reaction (PCR), a more sensitive and more specific technique than microscopy. It enables the detection of very low levels of parasitemia, and the precise identification of *Plasmodium* species.

In the most advanced countries, PCR is tending to become the reference method for recourse diagnosis (in situations of diagnostic difficulty). More rapid analysis methods, such as real-time PCR, are available in reference laboratories, and could be compatible with emergency or routine diagnosis.

2.3.9.2 Indirect diagnosis :

Serological method: The different techniques used are :

S Indirect immunofluorescence,

S Immunoelectrophoresis,

S Enzyme-linked immunosorbent assay (ELISA), These analytical techniques are not used for emergency diagnosis, but are useful for retrospective diagnosis of tropical fever, prevention of post-transfusion malaria, epidemiological surveys and monitoring of antibodies after an acute attack.

2.3.10 Management of malaria :

The management of malaria cases is a major component of malaria control strategies. Early diagnosis and prompt treatment with effective antimalarial drugs are essential for case management [52].

According to the National Malaria Control Programme (PNLP)

The programme's current recommendations are as follows

2.3.10.1 Malaria prevention methods

- The use of insecticide-impregnated mosquito nets for children and pregnant women
- IPT in pregnant women:

The drug of choice for IPT remains MS in pregnant women and other special groups (immunocompromised, sickle cell disease).

- Chemoprevention of seasonal malaria (CPS) in children aged 3 to 59 months
- Vector control :

Its aim is to reduce or even halt malaria transmission. It is based essentially on :

- Larval control: aimed at preventing or limiting the reproduction of mosquitoes.
- Rĕduction of human-vector contact: It must promote the use of

mosquito nets and curtains impregnated with insecticide, as well as spraying inside and outside the home.

- Environmental hygiene and sanitation: To destroy breeding grounds for anopheles and other mosquitoes.

2.3.10.2 Curative treatment of malaria :

1. Anti-malarial drugs

Anti-malarial drugs are chemically synthesised medicines or plant extracts designed to treat or prevent malaria.

Antimalarial drugs are classified according to their mode of action or chemical structure [54].

a. Erythrocyte schizonticide

Amino-alcohols: quinine (Quinimax®, Surquina®, Quinine Lafranc®), mefloquine (Lariam®), halofantrine (Halfan®), lumefantrine.

Amino-4-quinolines: chloroquine (Nivaquine®), amodiaquine (Flavoquine®), piperaquine.

Antimetabolites :

- Antifolates: sulphadoxine, dapsone,

- Antifolinics: proguanil (Paludrine®), pyrimethamine (Malocidea),
- Antibiotics: cyclins (Doxypalu®, Granudoxy®Ge, Vibraveineuse®), clindamycin (Dalacine®, Zindacine®),
- Ubiquinone analogues: atovaquone

Sesquiterpenes: artemisinin and its derivatives: dihydroartemisinin, artemether, artesunate

b.   Intrahepatic schizonticides :

- Amino 8 quinolines: primaquine (Primaquine®), tafenoquine.
- Antimëtabolites: proguanil, cyclins

   c.   Gametocytocides: Amino-8-quinolines: primaquine (Primaquine®), tafĕnoquine.

❖Amino-alcohols

> QUININE AND ITS DERIVATIVES :

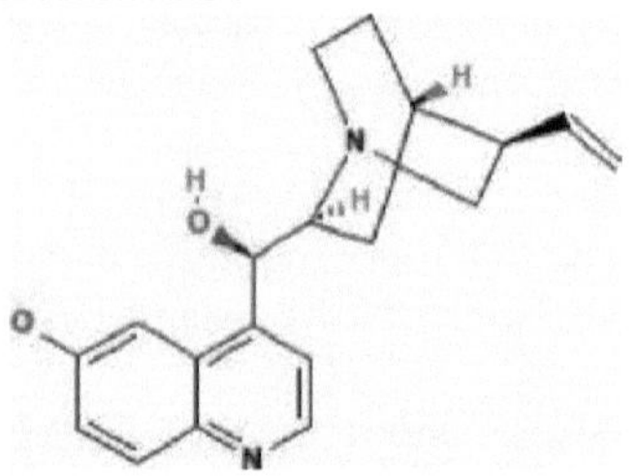

Figure 6: Chemical structure of quinine

<u>Source:</u>   https://pubchem.ncbi.nlm.nih.gov/compound/3034034#section=2D-Structure   (8a, 9R) -6'-Methoxycinchonan-9-ol trihydrate

NB: Any change in the chemical structure of quinine alters its pharmacological action.

Pharmacological properties

Quinine is a natural antimalarial with rapid schizonticidal activity in the blood against the various plasmodial species. It is a drug used to treat severe malaria, especially when infused intravenously. It has no activity on the gametes *P. Vivax, P. Ovale, P. malariae* are extremely sensitive to quinine. *P. falciparum* is generally sensitive, but some strains are resistant.

Mechanism of action

Like chloroquine, quinine concentrates in the digestive vacuole of Plasmodium, but at lower concentrations than chloroquine. As with mefloquine, binding to the parasite's protein sites may be favoured by the drug's lipophilicity. It is a product recommended for the treatment and prevention of malaria, even in chloroquine-resistant areas.

Pharmacokinetics

Absorption: rapid by the oral or intramuscular route.

Bioavailability: 80%. Half-life: 11 hours.

Mëtabolism: by CYP 3A4.

Elimination: renal, 20% in unchanged form, 80% in the form of metabolites, including an active metabolite, hence the need to adjust dosage in patients with renal insufficiency. The pharmacokinetics of quinine are significantly modified by malaria infection: quinine concentrations sometimes increase as a result of a reduction in the apparent volume of distribution and hepatic and renal clearance of quinine.

Undesirable effects

They are dose-dependent:

-Frequent, not very serious: cinchonism (tinnitus, dizziness, headache, blurred vision, acute hearing loss, digestive problems, peripheral vasodilatation).

-Hypoglycemia due to increased insulin secretion. Quinine is contraindicated in cases of cardiac rhythm disorders, history of bilious fever, haemoglobinuria, allergy to quinine, in association with astemizole-based medication (antiallergic).

Presentation and dosage

Quinine comes in the form of :

-300 mg, 125 mg and 500 mg tablets.

- Injectable ampoules with doses of 125 mg, 250 mg, 500 mg, 100 mg and 400 mg.

Quinine is administered at a dose of 8mg/kg/3 times/day for 7 days.

Quinidine :

It is even more effective against *P. falciparum* than quinine. It is not usually used because of its activity on cardiac conduction. However, it could be used if quinine is unavailable, subject to cardiac and electrical monitoring. Other cinchona alkaloids are less active.

> Lumefantrine

Lumefantrine is an antimalarial drug intended to treat uncomplicated Plasmodium falciparum malaria. It is always used in fixed combination with Artemether in an Artemether/lumefantrine ratio, as lumefantrine monotherapies are not approved anywhere in the world.

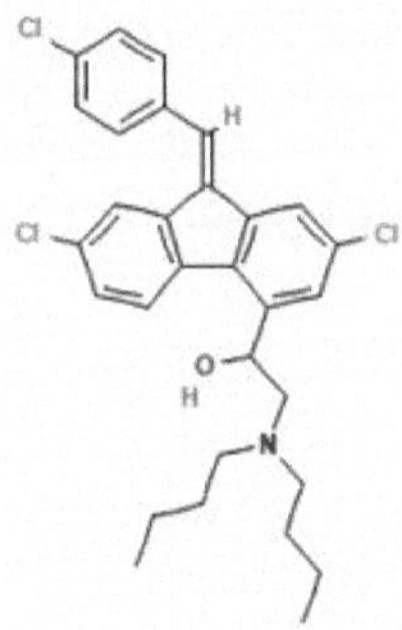

Figure 7: Chemical structure of Lumefantrine

2-(dibutylamino)-1-[(9Z)-2,7-dichloro-9-(4-chlorobenzylidene)-9H-fluoren-4-yl] ethanol

<u>Source</u> : https://pubchem.ncbi.nlm.nih.gov/compound/6437380#section=2D-Structure

Pharmacokinetics

Lumefantrine is a highly lipophilic molecule, and its absorption, which is greatly enhanced by the consumption of a fatty meal, begins approximately 2 hours after oral administration, with peak plasma concentration reached between 6 and 8 hours after administration. Its bioavailability varies and is high depending on whether the drug is administered with a fatty food. It is strongly bound to plasma lipoproteins. Lumefantrine is metabolised in animals by glucuroconjugation after oxidative biotransformation to desbutyl-lumefantrine, a metabolite whose in vitro antiparasitic effect is 5 to 8 times greater than that of Lumefantrine. Lumefantrine has an elimination half-life of 4 to 6 days in subjects infected with *P. falciparum*. It is always used in fixed combination with Artemether in a ratio of Artemether/I.umefantrine **[58]**.

Mechanism of action

It concentrates in the nutrient vacuole of Plasmodium, acting by binding to ferriprotoporphyrin IX and blocking its polymerisation into hemozoin (a pigment that is non-toxic to plasmodia).

❖ 4-AMINOQUINOLINES

4-aminoquinolines are organic compounds consisting of a quinoline molecule substituted in position 4 by an amino group. This amino-quinoline is the basis of certain antimalarial drugs.

Mechanism of action

Chloroquine, amodiaquine and piperaquine were the first synthetic antimalarial drugs, isolated between 1938 and 1941. Amino-4-quinolines are weak bases; they diffuse into the parasite's red blood cells, accumulating in the parasite's digestive vacuole and reducing its acidity. Digestion of haemoglobin (proteolysis) by the erythrocyte plasmodium releases ferriprotoporphyrin IX, which is toxic to the parasite. The parasite neutralises it by polymerisation into an insoluble pigment (hemozoin). These drugs block the detoxification of the heme by the parasite. As well as being erythrocytic schizonticide

Amodiaquine

Mono-desehylamodiaquine: 4-((7-Chloro-4-quinolinyl) amino)-2- ((Ethylamino) methyl) phenol

Formula: C18H18ClN3O

It is a 4-amino-quinoline whose mode of action is similar to that of chloroquine. After being abandoned in the 1980s, it regained interest ten years later in the treatment of simple acne. Ten years later, it gained renewed interest in the treatment of uncomplicated access. It is effective against certain chloroquine-resistant strains of *P. falciparum*, even if cross-resistance exists.

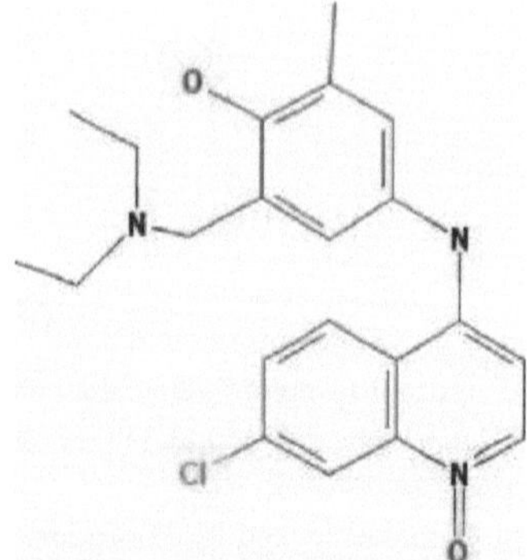

Figure 8: Chemical structure of Amodiaquine

Source : https://pubchem.ncbi.nlm.nih.gov/compound/2165#section=Top 4-[(7-chloro-4-quinolinyl) amino] -2-[(diethylamino)] methylphenol

Pharmaceutical forms

Comprimës containing 200 mg or 153.1 mg of amodiaquine base in hydrochloride form (Flavoquine®, Camoquin®)

Pharmacokinetics

Amodiaquine is rapidly absorbed after oral administration and mëtabolisëd at the hëpatic level by cytochrome P450 2C8 to the active metabolite desehylamodiaquine. Both amodiaquine and desehylamodiaquine are highly bound to plasma proteins (>90%). However, amodiaquine concentrations are much lower, and its elimination half-life much shorter than that of its metabolite (3 to 8 hours versus 8 days).

Mechanism of action

The pharmacodynamics are based on amodiaquine and desehylamodiaquine, which accumulate strongly in the parasitic digestive vacuole and exert a schizonticidal activity. This lysosomotropic activity consists of inhibiting the digestion of hemoglobin by plasmodia. They interfere with intra-parasitic polymerisation and alter the transformation of toxic heme, a toxic product resulting from the dëgradation of l'ЪётодloЬlne by the plasmodia, into hëmozoin (an insoluble, non-toxic pigment).

Indications: Treatment of uncomplicated plasmodium-sensitive malaria

Contraindications : The administration of amodiaquine is contraindicated:

- in subjects with known hypersensitivity^ to amodiaquine;
- in subjects suffering from hëpatic disorders;
- as chemoprophylaxis

Undesirable effects: The most common ëbeing nausea, vomiting, abdominal pain, diarrhoea and dëmangement. Eating disorders caused by amodiaquine are less frequent than with chloroquine.

Toxicity :

The main toxic effects of amodiaquine are l^patotoxic^ and severe agranulocytosis, sometimes fatal when the drug is used as chemoprophylaxis. This amodiaquine toxicity appears to be mediated by amodiaquine quinone imine, a metabolite with immunogenic properties derived from the oxidative metabolism of amodiaquine [57].

Amodiaquine toxicity may cause syncope, spasticity, convulsions and involuntary movements after taking high doses of amodiaquine.

❖ANTIMETABOLITES :

Les Antifoliques :

> Sulphonamides

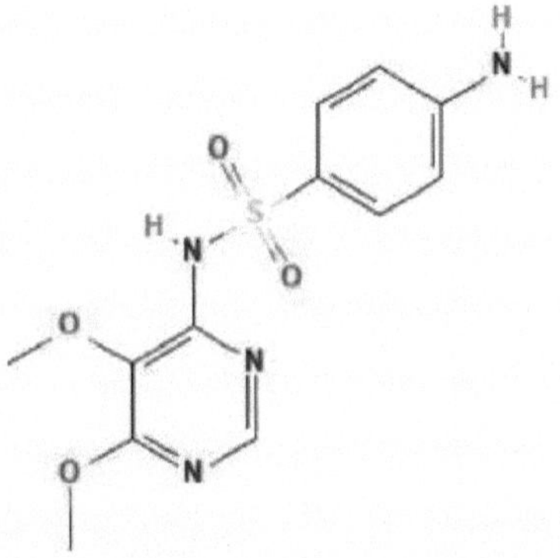

Figure 9: Chemical structure of Sulfadoxine

Source: https://pubchem.ncbi.nlm.nih.gov/compound/17134#section=2D-Structure 4-amino-

N-(5,6-dimethoxy-4-pyrimidinyl) benzenesulfonamide

- **Molecular weight: 310.3 (C12H14N4O4S)**

Sulphadoxine is a sulphonamide which is eliminated slowly. It is very slightly soluble in water. Sulphonamides are structural analogues and antagonists of p-aminobenzoic acid acting by compëtition. They are competitive inhibitors of dihydroptëroate synthëtase, the bacterial enzyme responsible for incorporating p-aminobenzoic acid into the synthesis of folic acid.

- **Formulations** : Sulfadoxine is used as a fixed combination of 20 parts sulfadoxine to 1 part pyrimethamine and can be administered orally or intramuscularly as :
-   tablets containing 500 mg sulfadoxine and 25 mg pyrimethamine;
-   ampoules containing 500 mg of sulfadoxine and 25 mg of pyrimethamine in 2.5 ml of solution for intramuscular injection.

- **Pharmacokinetics**: Sulphadoxine is rapidly absorbed from the digestive tract. Peak blood levels occur 4 hours after oral administration.

Its terminal elimination half-life is 4 to 9 days. Almost 90-95% of sulphadoxine is bound to plasma proteins. It is widely distributed in tissues and body fluids, passes into the ileal circulation and is found in breast milk. It is mainly excreted as such in the urine.

- Toxicity: Sulphadoxine shares the adverse effect profile of other sulphonamides, but may cause severe allergic reactions due to its slow elimination. Nausea, vomiting, anorexia and diarrhoea may occur. Crystalluria causing back pain, haematuria and oliguria are rare compared to other more rapidly eliminated sulphonamides. Hypersensitivity reactions may affect various organs. Skin manifestations may be severe and include pruritus, photosensitivity reactions, erythroderma, erythema nodosum, bullous erythroderma with epidermolysis, Stevens-Johnson syndrome and Lyell syndrome; Lyell syndrome is characterised by the sudden destruction and detachment of the superficial layer of the skin (epidermis) and mucous membranes (epithelium) over a large part of the body. Sulfadoxine treatment should be discontinued in any patient with a rash due to the risk of severe allergic reactions. Hypersensitivity to sulphadoxine may also cause interstitial nephritis, back pain, haematuria and oliguria. These are due to the formation of crystals in the urine (crystalluria) and can be avoided by keeping the patient well hydrated in order to maintain a high urine flow rate. Other adverse reactions reported include hypoglycaemia, icterus neonatorum, clear fluid meningitis, somnolence, fatigue, cephalalgia, ataxia, vertigo, convulsions, neuropathy, psychosis and ucomembranous enterocolitis.

Antifolinics

> Pyrimethamine :

Cl

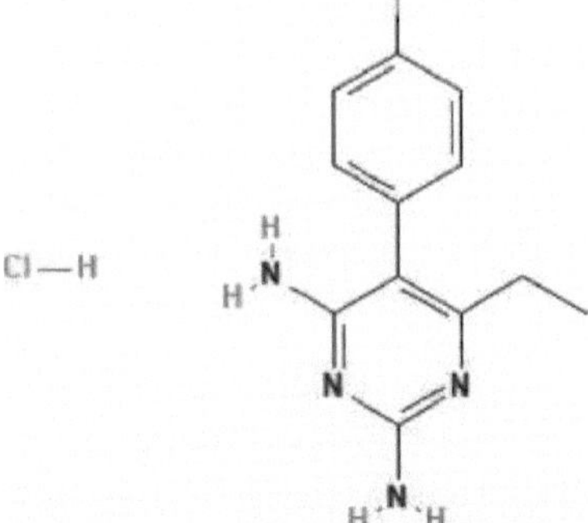

Figure 10: Chemical structure of pyrimethamine

5-(4-chlorophenyl)-6-ethyl-2,4-pyriminediamine
<u>Source</u> : https://pubchem.ncbi.nlm.nih.gov/compound/4993#section=2D-Structure
- **Molecular weight**: 248.7 (C12H13ClN4)

Pyrimethamine is a diaminopyrimidine used in combination with a sulfonamide, in дёпёгаl sulfadoxine or dapsone. It exerts its antimalarial activity by inhibiting plasmodial dihydrofolate reductase and thus indirectly blocking nucleic acid synthesis in hematozoa.

It is a slow-acting blood schizonticide that can also be active against pre-erythrocytic forms and inhibits the development of sporozoites in the mosquito vector. It is effective against all four types of malaria encountered in humans, even if resistance develops rapidly. Pyrimethamine is also used in the treatment of toxoplasmosis and isosporosis, and as a prophylactic against Pneumocystiscarinii pneumonia. Pyrimethamine is no longer used on its own as an antimalarial; it is only used in synergistic combination with slow-release sulphonamides for treatment (sulfadoxine, sulfalene) or with dapsone for prophylaxis.

Formulations

Pyrim6thamine is currently mainly етрloyёe in fixed combinations with slowly eliminating sulphonamides, for example 20 parts sulphadoxine to 1 part pyr^ё^т^, for which combination there are oral and parentëral formulations in the form of: - comprimës containing 500 mg of sulfadoxine and 25 mg of pyrimëthamine; - ampoules containing 500 mg of sulfadoxine and 25 mg of pyrimëthamine in 2.5 ml of injectable solution for the intramuscular route.

- **Pharmacokinetics**

Pyrimëthamine is almost completely absent from the digestive tract and peak plasma levels occur 2-6 hours after oral ingestion. It is mainly concentrated in the kidneys, lungs, liver and spleen and almost 80-90% of pyrimëthamine binds to plasma protëines. It is metabolised in the liver and slowly excreted by the kidneys. Its plasma half-life is approximately 4 days. Pyrimëthamine crosses the hëmato-encëphalic and placental barriers and is found in breast milk. Absorption of the intramuscular preparation is incomplete and not sufficiently reliable for this formulation to be recommended.

- **Toxicity**

Pyrimëthamine is generally well tolerated. Its administration for prolonged periods may cause matopoietic suppression due to its interference with the metabolism of folic acid. Skin rashes and hypersensitivity reactions may also occur. Larger doses may cause digestive symptoms such as dëpapillating glossitis, abdominal pain and vomiting, hëmatological effects including mëgaloblastic a^mia, leucopënia, thrombopënia and pancytopënia and central nervous system effects: cëphalëes and dizziness. Acute overdosage of pyrimëthamine may cause gastrointestinal effects and central nervous system stimulation with vomiting, excitability^ and convulsions, which may be followed by tachycardia, respiratory dëpression, cardiovascular collapse and dëces of the patient. In the event of an overdose, supportive treatment will be applied.

SESQUITERPENES: ARTEMISININ AND ITS DERIVATIVES
Artemisinin and its derivatives Artemisinin is a medicinal active substance extracted in 1972 by Chinese scientists from the Chinese medicinal plant Artemisia annua L (Qinghao). The plant's medicinal virtues were discovered in China over 2000 years ago, to reduce fever and relieve symptoms of malaria.

Artemisinin and its derivatives are sesquiterpene lactones which possess endo-peroxide bridges responsible for their schizonticidal properties.

The main derivatives are dihydro-artemisinin, artemether, artesunate and arteether. Artemisinin derivatives are active at all stages of the parasite's development, and are also gametocytocidal(64). Artemisinin and its derivatives, the 1,2,4-trioxanes, act rapidly and are highly active against erythrocytic parasites, but they have a short half-life (between 45 min and 3 h), which is why they should be combined with other antimalarial drugs with longer activity to form CTAs.

ACTs are effective against multi-resistant strains and, since 2006, have been the first-line treatment recommended by the WHO.

Artemether-lumefantrine and artesunate-amodiaquine are used as first-line artemisinin-based combination therapies in West Africa **[59]**.

Artemether combined with Lumefantrine, known as Coartem®, is the first high-quality ACT for children. Artesunate is the best drug for treating complicated and severe forms of malaria **[45]**. It is formulated for injection under the name Artesun® and is also combined with mefloquine (Artequin®), pyronaridine (Pyramax®) or amodiaquine (Coarsucam®). The combination of dihydroartemisinin with piperaquine is sold under the name Eurartesim® **[60]**.

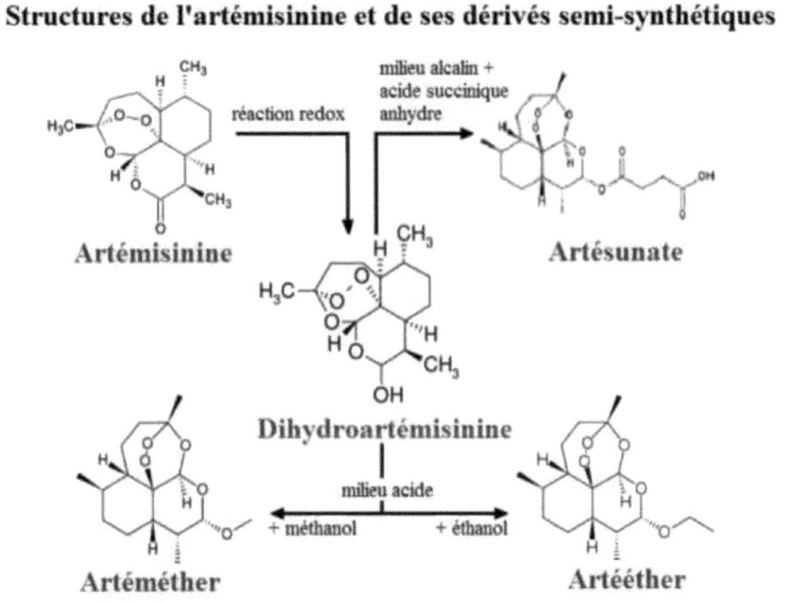

Figure 11: Rë structural action of CTAs.

Mechanism of action

Artemisinin is a sesquiterpene lactone bearing a peroxide group, which appears to be the clë of its efficacy. It is thought to block an enzyme that allows the parasite to pump calcium, thus preventing it from developing. Artemether, on the other hand, i.e. the reduced peroxide molecule in artemisinin, reacts with the iron in red blood cells to create free radicals which, in turn, destroy the membranes of the parasite or certain cancer cells and kill them. It should be noted, however, that the presence of any substance protecting against free radical damage (antioxidant) could counteract its effectiveness. Their active metabolite, dihydro-artemisinin, interacts with haemoglobin in the parasitophorous vacuole and causes the release of free radicals. These free radicals inhibit plasmodial protein synthesis, thereby blocking replication of the parasite's nucleic acids [45].

2. Simple malaria :

A patient presenting with one of the symptoms/signs of malaria (fever above 37°C, headache, fever, chills, muscle pain, aches, nausea, vomiting, sweating, etc.) combined with a positive RDT or EW/MF, according to NMCP guidelines, before treatment is started. Simple malaria is effectively treated orally. Artemisinin-based Combination Therapies (ACTs) are currently the recommended and most effective treatment.

They come in tablet and oral suspension forms.

They are effective in treating uncomplicated malaria in 3 days [61].

The WHO proposes five (CTA) which are :

- Artesunate + Mefloquine

- Artesunate + Sulfadoxine-Pyrimethamine
- Dihydroartemisin-piperaquine (DHA-PQ)
- Artemether + Lumefantrine (AL)
- Artesunate + Amodiaquine

The national malaria control programme recommends the following combinations for the treatment of malaria in Mali:

- Artemether + Lumefantrine (AL)
- Artesunate + Amodiaquine

The two artemisinin-based combinations were selected for the treatment of uncomplicated cases of malaria on the basis of the following criteria:

- therapeutic efficacy,
- clinical safety,
- acceptability and compliance with treatment,
- cost-effectiveness,
- ability to delay drug resistance,

availability and the possibility of widespread geographical use.

Table 2: Presentation and dosage of Artemether 20 mg - Lumefantrine 120 mg, tablet (CP)

Weight / Age groups	Day 1		Day 2		Day 3	
	Morning	Evening	Morning	Evening	Morning	Evening
05-14Kg(2months3years)	lcp	lcp	lcp	lcp	lcp	lcp
15-24 Kg (4 to 6 years old}	2cp	2cp	2cp	2cp	2cp	2cp
25-34 kg(7a IDans)	3cp	3cp	3cp	3cp	3cp	3cp
> 35 Kgetadultes	4cp	4cp	4cp	4cp	4cp	4cp

Table 3: АЛётёЛег 180+ Lumëfantrine 1080mg suspension 60ml

Child's weight	Number of millilitres		
	1er day	2eme day	3eme day
5 to 9 kg (6-11 months)	10ml	10ml	10ml
10 to 15 kg (1-3 years)	20ml	20ml	20ml

Table 4: Presentation and dosage of artesunate-amodiaquine

Weight range (Age range	Presentation	1er treatment day	2eme day of treatment	3eme day of treatment
>4.5kg a < 9kg (2 months)	25mg/67.5mg pack of 3cp	1cp	1cp	1cp
>9kg to <18kg (l allans)	50 mg/135 mg Blister of 3cp	1cp	1cp	1cp
>18kg a <36kg (6 al3years)	100 mg/270 mg Blister of 3cp	1cp	1cp	1cp
> 36kg (l4 years and over)	100 mg/270 mg Blister of 6cp	2cp	2cp	2cp

NB: the first dose must be taken under supervision. If the child vomits within 30 minutes, repeat the dose.

What to do if signs persist :

It is important to re-examine the patient and repeat the biological diagnosis.

If the patient has followed the treatment correctly and the biological test is positive:
Look for other causes of fiëvre or refer for ëvaluation If treatment is not followed,
Resume treatment under medical supervision. If laboratory tests cannot be carried out,
Rëfërer to a higher level.

Adjuvant treatment Drugs and dosage to be administered :
Paracdtamol 500 mg: 15 to 20 mg/kg every 6 hours;
Iron 200mg: 2 tablets/day (adult) or 10 mg/kg/day (child) if andmia ;
Folic acid 5mg: Icomprimds/day if andmia
❖ Advice for patients
When can I return immediately?
If the fever persists;
If the child finds it difficult to drink and unable to eat;
If convulsion (ocular rdvulsion) ;
If unable to sit ;
If vomiting persists;
If becomes unconscious ;
If heat or ictere ;
If there is blood in the stools
If dark urine ;
If breathing difficulties
Focus on :
S Follow-up visit after 3 days of treatment if symptoms persist;
S The need to continue feeding;
S Continue to take the drug even if the patient is feeling better;
S Malaria prevention (use of long-lasting insecticide-impregnated mosquito nets for children and pregnant women, IPT for pregnant women and CPS for children aged between 3 and 59 months);
S Extensive use of CSCom for later episodes

3. Severe malaria :
Patients with signs of uncomplicated malaria associated with one or more of the following: prostration, recurrent convulsion, loss of consciousness, respiratory distress, severe hypoglycaemia (< 1.2 ml/l), severe anaemia (haemoglobin < 5 g/dl or haematocrit < 15%), cardiovascular collapse and shock.
The main aim of treating severe malaria is to prevent death. The prevention of neurological sequelae is an important component of the treatment of neuromalaria. In pregnant women, the main aim of malaria treatment is to save the life of the mother and the foetus **[53]**.
•   **CSCom/CSRef/Hospital levels :**
Treatment is based on two essential ëléments:
•   Emergency treatment of complications: which is vital for the patient. The onset of dëcës may be due to the disease itself or to its complications.
•   Specific antimalarial treatment: this is essential and extremely urgent, and must be administered very quickly to stop the disease spreading further.
•   **Emergency treatment of complications :**
These are symptomatic treatments aimed at correcting hypoglycëmia, dëshydration, afemia, lowering fever, stopping convulsions and managing coma and respiratory, renal and

cardiovascular problems.

S **Treatment of hypoglycaemia :**

In children and adolescents, administer slowly by IV:

- 3 to 5 ml /kg for sërum glucosë at 10% or
- 1 ml/kg for 30% sërum glucosë.

S **For adults, administer slowly by IV :**

- 3 to 5 ml /kg for sërum glucosë 10% or
- 1 ml/kg for 30% sërum glucosë or
- 25 ml of 50% sërum glucosë : If you only have 50% sërum glucosë, dilute one part of it with a little water.

volume in 4 volumes of sterile water to obtain a 10% solution (for example, 0.4 ml/kg of 50% glucosë with 1.6 ml/kg of water for injections or 4 ml of 50% glucosë with 16 ml of water for injections). Hypertonic glucosë (> 20%) is not recommended as it has an irritant effect on the përiphëric veins. When intravenous administration is not possible, give glucose or any other sugar solution through a nasogastric tube.

S **Treatment of dehydration**

- Administer 100 ml/kg of lactated Ringer's solution over 2 or 4 hours,
- Rëë assess the patient afterwards to determine water requirements and the state of dehydration.

Treatment of convulsions

- Administer diazëpam at a dose of 0.5 mg/kg intra rectally (IR) or IM,
- If convulsions persist 10 to 15 mg / kg phënobarbital parenterally.

Treatment of anemia :

- In case of sëvëre anemia (hemoglobin level < 5g/dl): emergency blood transfusion: 20 ml /kg of whole blood for 4 hours on furosemide or 10 ml /kg of packed red blood cells in children.
- If transfusion is impossible: carry out pre-transfer treatment before sending the patient to a centre with a blood transfusion service.

In case of coma :

- Assess the stage of coma (Blantyre or Glasgow scale),
- Place the patient in a lateral safety position,
- Aspirates secretions and clears the airways,
- Insert a nasogastric feeding tube,
- Take a venous line,
- Place a urinary catheter,
- Change the patient's position every 4 hours,
- Measure urine volume (diuresis).

In the event of breathing difficulties: (Acute Lung Injury)

- Put the patient in a semi-seated position, administer furosemide IV: 2 to 4 mg/kg and Гохудёие
- Check that he does not have heart failure due to sevëre anemia,
- If possible, evacuate the patient to an intensive care unit.

In case of renal insufficiency :

- Administer solutions if the patient is dehydrated: 20ml/kg isotonic saline serum, 1 to 2 mg/kg furosemide,

- Place a bladder catheter,
- If the patient does not pass urine within 24 hours,
- Transfer to a centre for dialysis.

N.B: other serious illnesses must be treated in accordance with the appropriate scheme.

- **Specific antimalarial treatment**

Severe malaria can be treated with :

> **Artesunate** is the médicament of choice for the treatment of severe malaria. It can be administered as an intravenous (IV) or intramuscular (IM) injection. Aresunate 2.4 mg/kg body weight administered intravenously (IV) or intramuscularly (IM) on admission (H = 0), then H12 and H24 later and, thereafter, once daily for no more than 7 days, for patients weighing 20 kg or more.

For children weighing less than 20kg: artesunate 3mg/kg bodyweight at the times indicated above.

Procedure for diluting Artesunate :

IV route: a vial containing 60 mg of Artesunate will be diluted with 1 ml of sodium bicarbonate and 5 ml of sodium chloride, so that the final solution contains 10 mg/ml of Artesunate.

IM route: the 60 mg vial of Artesunate powder will be diluted with 1 ml of sodium bicarbonate and 2 ml of sodium chloride, so that the final solution contains 20 mg/ml of Artesunate.

- Detach the top of the Artesunate bottle and disinfect the rubber using 10% povidone-iodine or an alcohol swab.
- Open the two ampoules of bicarbonate and sodium chloride beforehand so that you can hold the syringe with the needle in your hands during the process.
- Draw 1 ml of 5% sodium bicarbonate into a syringe and inject it into the Artesunate bottle.
- Shake until the Artesunate powder has completely dissolved and the solution is clear. Do not shake too vigorously to avoid the formation of foam on the surface of the solution. If the solution is cloudy or there is a precipitate, the parenteral preparation should be discarded.
- The needle is withdrawn backwards so that it is no longer in contact with the liquid and the air jet is removed from the vial to ensure there is sufficient space in the vial to inject the dilution solution.

NB: Never use l'eau distilMe or l'eau physiologique to dilute I'Art^sunate because water for injection is not a diluent appropпë.

- Draw 5 ml of the 0.9% sodium chloride into a syringe and inject into the vial of Artësunate for the IV route. Withdraw 2 ml of the 0.9% sodium chloride into a syringe and inject it into the bottle of Artësunate for the IM route.
- Remove the required volume of Artësunate from the vial (according to the dosage sclwma). Discard any excess solution.
- The solution is administered slowly by IV over 2 to 3 minutes.

The routes of administration are direct IV or IM. If injectable Artësunate is not available, it can be replaced by Artëmëther or quinine.

- **Artemether injection IM**

Dosage and administration

Intramuscular treatment over 5 days:

The dosage is 3.2mg/kg body weight in one injection on admission, followed by 1.6mg/kg in one injection per day.

Table 5: Dosage and administration of Artëmëther in children aged 0 - 5 years: 20 mg ampoules.

Age	Weight	Day 1	Day 2	Day 3	Day 4	Day 5
< 1 year	5 - 9 Kg	1 amp	½ amp	½ amp	½ amp	½ amp
2 - 5 years	10 - 15 Kg	2 amp	1 amp	1 amp	1 amp	1 amp

Table 6: Dosage and administration of Artemether in subjects over 5 years of age: 80 mg ampoules.

Age	Weight	Day 1	Day 2	Day 3	Day 4	Day 5
6 - 13 years	16 - 35 Kg	1 amp	½ amp	½ amp	½ amp	½ amp
14 years and over more	> 35 kg	2 amp	1 amp	1 amp	1 amp	1 amp

<u>Source</u>: National guidelines for the management of malaria cases in Mali 2016 Take over with oral ACTs as soon as the patient can swallow them.

> Quinine injection (infusion or IM).

Recommended dosage

Quinine is administered by slow intravenous (IV) infusion mixed in a solutë

Loading dose: 20 mg quinine salt/kg) on admission in adults and children

Maintenance dose

Adult: 10 mg/kg of quinine salts (8.3 mg base) diluted in 10 ml/kg of a hypertonic solution infused over 4 hours with 10% glucose, 4.3% dextrose or (0.9% isotonic saline serum for diabetics).

- Interval between the start of infusions: 8 hours,
- Infusion time: 4 hours.
- The duration of treatment with quinine is seven (7) days.

NB: take quinine tablets with sugar water to prevent hypoglycaemia.

Intramuscular (IM) quinine If administration by intravenous (IV) infusion is not possible, then give the same dose (10 mg/kg) intra-muscularly (IM) every 8 hours and continue until the patient is able to take the treatment orally. The injection should be made into the anterolateral aspect of the thigh. Give the patient sugar water to prevent hypoglycaemia.

Note: IM injections must be made as aseptically as possible in the antero-external aspect of the thigh in children and not in the buttock.

Switch to the oral route using CTAs as soon as the patient's condition allows.

4. Treatment of malaria in pregnant women

The drug for intermittent preventive treatment (IPT) is still Sulfadoxine Pyrimethamine (SP), which is recommended to prevent malaria during pregnancy. The WHO recommends a schedule of at least four prenatal consultations during pregnancy. It is recommended that IPT-

SP be administered at all scheduled antenatal visits from the beginning of the second trimester.

Insecticide-treated mosquito nets should be provided as early as possible in the first trimester. A single dose is given as three tablets (500 mg Sulfadoxine and 25 mg pyrimethamine per tablet), administered under direct observation. IPTg-SP should be administered to all pregnant women, but only at the start of the second trimester.

The following doses must be administered at each prenatal contact at least 4 weeks apart.

The last dose can be administered right up to the moment of delivery without posing a safety problem.

When should I avoid giving MS?

- Ask the woman if she has any allergies to sulphonamides, including SP, before administering it. If she is allergic to sulphonamides, do not give her SP; focus on IBD and other preventive measures.

- Do not give MS to women during the first trimester of pregnancy.

- Do not administer SP to pregnant women taking folic acid at a daily dose of > 5 mg, as this neutralises the effectiveness of its antimalarial action. The WHO recommends a daily dose of folic acid of 0.4 mg during pregnancy.

- Women taking cotrimoxazole for the treatment of other infections (e.g. seropositive women) should not take SP.

- Do not give MS if the woman has taken it in the last 4 weeks.

Malaria is serious in pregnant women, with a twofold risk:

- risk of severe stroke in the mother.

- risk to the foetus: spontaneous abortion or premature delivery.

Any malaria infection in a pregnant woman should therefore be treated as a matter of urgency with quinine (the only drug that can be used). However, it should be borne in mind that the risk of hypoglycaemia during *P. falciparum* infection, *which is* increased by quinine, is more frequent in pregnant women.

> **Simple malaria**

First trimester of pregnancy: quinine salt comprrimë at a dose of 10mg/kg every 8 hours for 7 days.

Second and third trimesters of pregnancy: CTA

> **Severe malaria**

Artesunate is the treatment of choice. If this drug is unavailable, Artëmëther is preferable to quinine in late pregnancy, as quinine is associated with a 50% risk of hypoglycaemia.

NB: Switch to the oral route as soon as the patient can swallow (Quinine tablet for pregnant women in the first trimester of pregnancy and CTA from the second trimester of pregnancy).

2.3.11 Means of preventing and controlling malaria

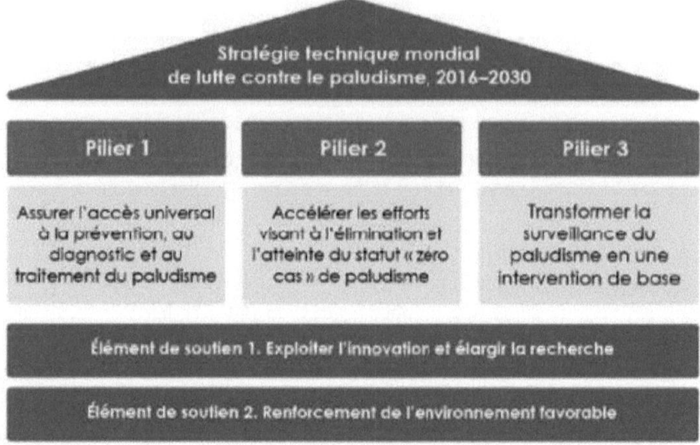

Figure 12: The three pillars of the Global Technical Strategy for Malaria Control
(Source: WHO, 2015)

Efforts to control and prevent malaria focus essentially on reducing contact between humans and mosquitoes, reducing the number of people infected, and reducing the mosquito population through vector control measures.

The most effective strategies used worldwide are :

- The   vector control,
- The   Chemoprevention,
- Case management,
- Malaria   surveillance.

Vector control prevents mosquitoes from acquiring or transmitting infection through the use of insecticide-treated nets (ITNs) or long-lasting insecticide-treated nets (LLINs) and indoor residual spraying (IRS).

Chemoprevention suppresses and prevents infections in humans through intermittent preventive treatment for pregnant women (IPT) and seasonal chemoprevention (SCP).

Finally, case management detects, diagnoses, treats and cures infections using effective diagnostic tests and treatments. The combination of interventions may vary according to the specific context of each country.

Malaria surveillance detects and examines all malaria infections in order to prevent secondary infections.

Insecticide-treated mosquito nets : Insecticide-treated nets (ITNs) and long-lasting insecticide-treated nets (LLINs) reduce human-mosquito contact by drawing a protective barrier between mosquitoes and humans during the evening, when mosquitoes are usually feeding. When used correctly and consistently, ITNs reduce all-cause mortality by 17% and the number of malaria cases by 50%. The main difference between ITNs and LLINs is that LLINs are effective for at least 3 years, while ITNs are generally effective for 12 months.

Indoor residual **spraying** involves spraying the interior walls and ceilings of houses with insecticides to reduce human-mosquito contact. When the coverage rate of indoor residual spraying is high, the whole community is better protected, including households whose homes have not been sprayed.

Intermittent preventive treatment

Intermittent preventive treatment for pregnant women involves giving all pregnant women a dose of an antimalarial drug (currently sulfadoxine-pyrimethamine) during pregnancy to prevent and control malaria. It is recommended that IPT be given to pregnant women during routine antenatal visits at the beginning of the second trimester and doses should be taken at least 1 month apart [62].

Seasonal chemoprevention

The aim is to prevent infection during periods of high transmission by administering the SP+AQ (sulfadoxine-pyrimethamine + amodiaquine) combination to children aged between 3 and 59 months, every month, for a maximum of 4 doses. In most countries, these drugs are distributed mainly door-to-door [63].

Management of malaria cases

Effective management of malaria requires access to diagnostic tests and timely, effective treatment. Rapid parasitological confirmation either by microscopy or rapid diagnostic tests is recommended in all patients suspected of having malaria before treatment is started. Rapid and effective treatment involves receiving antimalarial treatment within the first 24 hours after the onset of malaria symptoms. The best treatment available to date, particularly for malaria caused by Plasmodium falciparum, is the artemisinin-based combination therapy, commonly known as ACT.

Malaria surveillance

Surveillance has been adopted as a fully-fledged malaria control intervention. Its aim is to detect all malaria infections, investigate every case of infection and ensure that every case detected is treated promptly to prevent secondary infections. Surveillance makes it possible to monitor diseases and respond programmatically, while taking decisions on the basis of the data collected.

Malaria vaccines

Malaria vaccines such as RTS, S/AS01 (RTS, S) and R21 Matrix-M are currently recommended by the WHO to prevent malaria in young children in Africa. They are active against *P. falciparum,* the most deadly parasite worldwide and also the most common in Africa. Malaria vaccines must be administered according to a 4-dose schedule to children from the age of 5 months.

In view of the potential public health benefits of the vaccine, the WHO's main advisory bodies on malaria and immunisation have jointly recommended its gradual introduction in selected areas of sub-Saharan Africa.

❖ Health indicators :

They are now an integral part of epidemiology in the broadest sense. They are used to measure health status using numerical indices, some of which are complex and based on a number of factors. They are complemented by risk indicators, the aim of which is to predict future events on the basis of observed criteria.

An indicator is a measure that summarises a set of statistics or serves as an indirect measure when information is not available. It assesses an element of a situation by describing its state or its evolution from a quantitative point of view. There are generally four categories of health indicator:

- **Socio-demographic indicators:** these give a general picture of the population and its socioeconomic level. They are useful for determining health and service needs.
- **Health indicators**: these measure the state of health of a population in terms of mortality and morbidity.

❖ **Malaria, indicators and indices**.

Malaria measurement assesses the intensity of malaria endemicity. It assesses the frequency and distribution of malaria within a given population. It can be used to define the different levels of transmission and endemicity, enabling malaria control strategies to be adapted to the biotope in question.

Malaria and indicators.

We can distinguish among others and according to their interest:

- Those assessing plasmodial infection:

Prevalence rate of plasmodial infections

Prevalence rate of placental plasmodial infections.

- Those who appreciate malaria morbidity:

Incidence rate of uncomplicated malaria: This is the rate of episodes of fever associated with clinical manifestations attributed to uncomplicated malaria.

Severe malaria incidence rate: This is the rate of clinical manifestations attributed to severe malaria.

Proportion of severe forms of malaria.

Prevalence of low birth weight

❖ **Indices in men**:

- Plasmodium index (PI): This is the percentage of subjects in a given age group (2 to 9 years) carrying asexual forms in peripheral blood. It is used to determine the level of endemicity. When the disease is known in the region and the number of cases is expected, given the place, time and population considered, there are 4 levels (percentage of the population): less than 25%: hypo-endemic; 25 to 50%: meso-endemic; 50 to 75%: hyper-endemic; more than 75%: holo-endemic.
- Splenic index: This is the percentage of children aged between 2 and 9 with splenomegaly. This index allows classification into hypo-endemic areas (splenic index from 0 to 19%), meso-endemic areas (splenic index from 20 to 49%), hyper-endemic areas (splenic index from 50 to 75%) and holo-endemic areas (splenic index greater than 75%). It is no longer used today.
- Gametocyte index: This represents the percentage of subjects carrying gametocytes in their blood. It indicates the capacity of a human population to infest vectors and therefore the risk of infectivity of a given population.
- **Evidence from the vector:** The importance of the role of anopheles in transmission is assessed by three indicators:

- Sporozoite index (SI): This is the percentage of anopheles carrying sporozoites in the salivary glands.
- Oocyst index (OI): This is the percentage of anopheles carrying oocysts in their stomach lining. This index is not very reliable because sporogonic involution can abort after oocyst formation.
- Entomological inoculation rate: The entomological inoculation rate or EIR represents the

number of infesting bites for humans and per ииПё of time. This ииПё can be expressed in nights, months or aniK'e according to the ёtudes entomologiques rёalisёes.

41

3 METHODOLOGY

3.1 Study location and framework :

Notre étude a ële realisee en commune I du District de Bamako au quartier Mekin-Sikoro au CSCOM, ce qui apparut important de faire un apergu général sur cette localite.

THEORETICAL HEALTH MAP OF THE MUNICIPALITY I

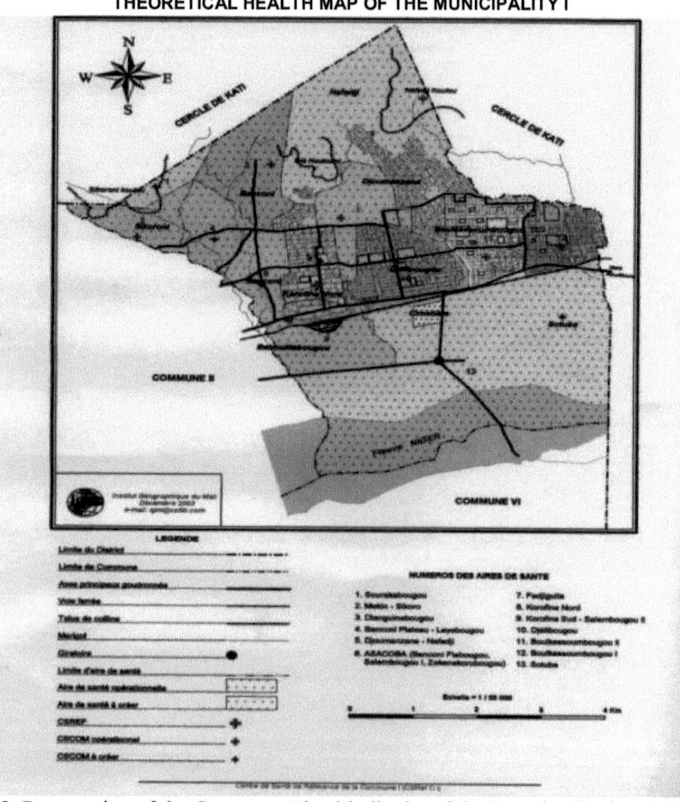

Figure 13: Presentation of the Commune I health district of the Bamako district

Presentation of the Mekin-Sikoro district :

M®kin-Sikoro covers an area of 9.39 km^2 . The district is bounded to the east by Banconi, to the north by Dialakorodji, to the south by the Hippodrome and to the west by N'Gomi.

The Mekin-Sikoro district comprises seven (07) sectors.

-     SikoroBase
-     SikoroPlateau
-     SikoroFeres
-   Sikoro   Faranida
-   Sikoro   Papre
-   Sikoro   Resettlement
-   Sikoro   Bamon

HISTORY :

Mekin-Sikoro is the oldest neighbourhood in the district, around which the village of Bamako was once built by the Niare people. It takes its name from a tree called "SI", which means karit®. The founder of the village of M®kin-Sikoro, Diamoussadjan Niare, is said to have come from Lambidou Soma Niakat® in the cercle of Di®ma. During a hunting trip, he discovered a site containing three karit® plants. He hung his bag on the first plant, his weapons of war on the second and went to sit under the third. Attracted by this place, he decided to found a village. Long before, he settled in Mekin®, 6 km from the uncovered site, and then in Ginkoum®, leaving his children behind in M®kin. According to the local authorities, Djamoussadjan Niar® would occasionally spend a year in M®kin-Sikoro before joining his children in M®kin and Tomo, where he also settled for a while. In fact, it was Djamoussadjan Niar®'s great-grandsons who finally settled in M®kin-Sikoro, giving it village status. According to history, all the Niar® of Bamako originated from M®kin-Sikoro, which at the time was considered to be the centre of power. Since its creation, the M®kin-Sikoro district has had eight (8) chiefs who have succeeded each other as chiefs, namely :

- Kamory Niar® 1st district chief r®gna for: 37 years
- S®riba Niar®: 40 years old
- Boh Niar®: 30 years

Bakoroba Niare: 35 years old
- Bandiougou Niare: 27 years old
- Balte Niare: 7 years
- Mamadou Niare : 1970-2021 :51 years dëcëdë on 20/08/21
- Flakoro Niare: (since October 2022)

In Mëкт-Sikoro the succession to chieftaincy is patriarchal.

3.2 Presentation of the Mekin-Sikoro ComHC

a.   Creation :

The Centre de Santë Communautaire de Mëкт-Sikoro is the fruit of a happy coopëration of the O.N. G -IAMANEH-SUISSE. It was officially ëlë cтëë on 08 March 1993. Its area of operation covers the Mëкт-Sikoro district. Also it benefits the populations of other districts.

b.   Composition

The ComHC comprises :

- Three (03) curative consultation rooms, one of which is ийНзëе for on-call duty
- Five (05) rooms for PN-PTME, CPON, declaration, PEV-CPES, PF and cervical cancer screening
- One (01) delivery room,
- One (01) 6-bed nappy room
- One (01) maternity ward^.
- One (01) 9-bed observation room for patients
- One (01) treatment room (injections and dressings),
- One (01) laboratory,
- One (01) daytime sales dëpбt,
- One (01) sales dëpбt for custody,
- One (01) shed for the EPI,
- One (01) shop at the maternity hospital^,
- One (01) room for CVD
- Two (02) toilet blocks for staff,

- One (01) block of two latrines for patients,

- One (01) latrine for patients.

Upstair

s we have :

2   A meeting room

3   An ultrasound   room

4   Unetoilette

5   A pharmacy for ARVs

6   An office for the chairman

7   Two offices for accountants, one of which is раЛадё with the management соткё

3.3 Organisation of the Mekin-Sikoro ComHC :

The CSCOM staff is made up of technical support staff (including three Doctors, a ^й^ёre d'Etat, a Biologist, seven Midwives, two Laborantines, a Matron, Two Nurse obstëtricians a Gërante du dëpбt de vente, two Accountants, a Caretaker, a Pharmacist for ARV), It is organisedë as follows:

- The Mëdecin Directeur is in charge of the centre and provides consultations, treatment for common illnesses and support management.

- The doctor in charge of reproductive health provides consultations and supervises the activities of the maternity unit. The third doctor provides curative consultations.

- The seven midwives provide childbirth, prenatal consultations, family planning, post-natal consultations and vaccinations.

- The Nurse assists the Doctor and provides medical care.

- The Biologist and Laboratory Technicians carry out laboratory analyses.

- The sales depot manager is responsible for selling the medicines.

- Obstetric nurses provide obstetric care and deliver babies.

- The Matron assists the midwives and also provides vaccinations and on-call duty;

- The Custodian ensures the security of the property.

-The housekeepers are responsible for hygiene, cleaning the premises and maintaining the CSCOM courtyard.

-Trainees.

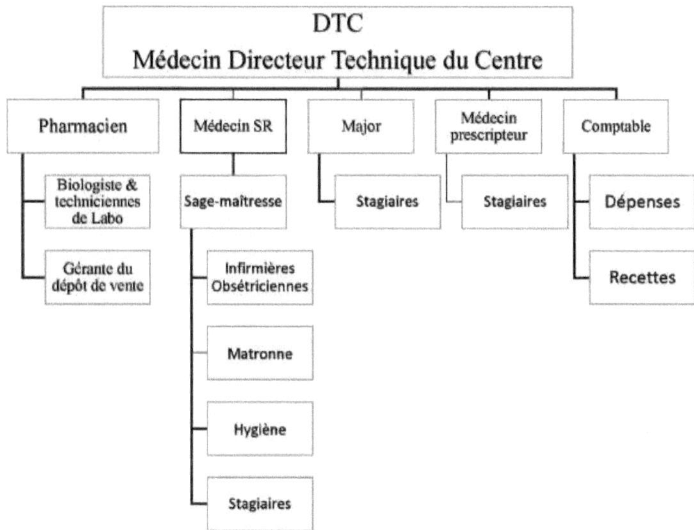

Figure 14: Organisation chart of the CSCom of Мёкт-Sikoro.

3.4 ComHC activities :

The ComHC's activities are as follows:

a. Curative :
-   consultations (curative, prenatal, postnatal, etc.);
-   childbirth ;
-   care (injections, infusions, dressings, sutures, etc.);
-   the fight against HIV/AIDS, malaria and other diseases.
-   Comprehensive care for HIV-positive adults and children

b. Preventive measures :
-   vaccination of children in the Expanded Programme on Immunization before the age of one (1) year;
-   vaccination of pregnant women and women of childbearing age with Tëtanus toxoid;
-   Prenatal consultations;

-   Postnatal consultations;
-   childbirth ;
-   preventive supervision of children from zëro (0) to twenty-three (23) months ;
-   regular monitoring of chronically ill patients and people at risk ;
-   Family planning.
-   vaccination against COVID-19

c. Promotional

Concerns :
•   Information, Education and Communication in Health (IECS);
•   promoting hygiene and sanitation activities ;
•   promoting community development activities.

d. Paraclinical examination activities :

45

- Blood: thick drop (GE), TDR, diagnostic serology phelix de Widal, glycemia, Urea, Creatinemia, HBs Antigen, serology BW, TE, Hb, Grouping/Rhesus;

serology -toxoplasmosis ; stool POK ; HIV serology and typing ;
- Urine: HCG test, ECBU; albuminuria, glucosuria;
- Sputum: BAAR are currently being analysed at the CSCOM;

The COVID-19 rapid diagnostic test

Ultrasound.

3.5 Management mechanism :

The CSCOM represents the technical operational unit of ASCOMSI. The ASACO is managed by two bodies democratically set up by the General Assembly:

The Board of Directors and the Management Committee. Like all other ComHCs, its operations are based on human, material and financial resources.

> **The Board of Directors:** The Board of Directors is the management body of the ComHC. Its members are elected by the General Assembly from among the members. It meets every three months in ordinary session and may meet in extraordinary session.

It exercises the powers necessary to implement the policy defined by the General Assembly. It exercises the powers necessary for the execution of the policy defined by the General Meeting.

In this capacity, it is responsible for :
- To convene ordinary and extraordinary meetings of the General Meeting, which shall be chaired by its Chairman:
- Proposing the ComHC's annual programme of activities and budget to the General Assembly
- Communicates the decisions of the General Assembly to the Management Committee and ensures that they are implemented. The Management Board is made up of two representatives from each locality and district in the health area.

> **The Management Committee**: The Management Committee is the body responsible for the day-to-day running of the Centre de Santë Communautaire's annual programme. Its members are ёlиз by the General Assembly in the same way as the Management Board. It meets in ordinary session once a month and may ёgalement meet in extraordinary session if necessary.

Its remit is to :
- Keep the ComHC's accounting records;
- Order, carry out or delegate and justify ;
- Approving, executing and receiving orders for medicines and supplies drawn up by the custodian and approved by the Head of Station;
- Ensuring the maintenance and repair of buildings and equipment;
- Prepares and submits to the management board the centre's annual activity report, programme and budget. The Management Committee is made up of six (6) members, including the Head of Post.

> **ComHC resources**: ComHC resources consist of revenue generated by :
- Curative, pre- and post-natal consultations;
- Childbirth ;
- Vaccinations ;

- Care ;
- The sale of mĕdicaments ;
- The sale of membership cards.

3.6 Type of study :

This was a cross-sectional study based on the use of clinical and laboratory consultation registers at the Mekin-Sikoro CSCOM during 2021 and interviews with malaria patients in 2022 on the use of malaria prevention methods (LLINs, IPTs, SPCs).

3.7 Study period :

The study focused on register data from 1er January to 31 December 2021 from the Mekin-sikoro CSCOM. Malaria patients were interviewed in October 2022.

3.8 The study population :

Our study concerned all people seen in consultation at the Mekin-Sikoro CSCOM during the year 2021 who had had a thick drop or a RDT (Rapid Diagnostic Test for malaria), and a sample of patients suffering from malaria in 2022 were also questioned about the use of anti-malaria measures.

3.9 Inclusion criteria

All people seen in consultation at the Mekin-Sikoro community health centre during 2021 who have had a thick drop or a malaria RDT.

3.10 Non-inclusion criteria

Patients seen in consultation who did not have a thick drop or RDT for malaria during the year 2021.

3.11 Sample size and Sampling

In view of the availability of registers and the time available, we carried out a sampling covering the year 2021 for the use of routine data from the ComHC.

The sample size for the work on malaria control measures is 234 for the interview, obtained using Daniel Schwartz's formula:

$$n = Z\alpha^2 \frac{pq}{i^2}$$

n: sample size

Z: parameter Hë at risk of error, Z = 1.96 for a risk of error of 5%.

P: Prevalence of malaria in Bamako according to EIP, 2021

q : Non-sick people p :1-P

i: precision fixed at 5%.

P= 3375 / 18059= 0,186 en 2021

$$n = 3,8416 \cdot \frac{(0,186 \times 1 - P)}{(0,05)^2} = 233,6 \approx 234$$

3.12 Variables measured

Use of registers

The information gathered covered :

- Patient identification (sociodëmographic)

> Name

> First name

> Age

> Gender

> Ethnic group

> Profession

> Rësidence

- Clinical :

Simple malaria

> Fever, Chills, Cëphalëe, Skin rash, Aches and pains, Abdominal pain, Nausea, Vomiting, Anorexia, Asthenia, Insomnia, Weight loss, Cough/cold, Diarrhea, Dizziness

Severe malaria

> Convulsion, severe anaemia, prostration,

- Parasitology

> Parasitemia

> Rapid Diagnostic Test (RDT),

- Treatment compliance

A treatment was considered correct if the choice of molecule, dosage, method of administration and duration complied with the recommendations of the national malaria control programme in Mali.

3.13 Operational definitions

Method for diagnosing malaria: set of procedures or tools used to confirm malaria.

Therapeutic regimen: set of methods for using medicines (route, form, dosage and duration of treatment).

3.14 Conduct of the study

Use of clinical registers

Six (6) clinical consultation registers were used to collect data from patients seen in consultation who had undergone the biological confirmation test (GE or RDT) for clinical malaria notified during the survey period (from 1er January to 31 December 2021). Approximately 86 incomplete records (1.28%) were rejected in order to obtain reliable results.

Use of laboratory registers

Three (3) Laboratory registers were used to collect certain information (socio-demographic data, additional examinations and their results (Qualitative and Quantitative).

This information did not always include age, place of residence or the result of the analysis.

Interviewing malaria patients

To carry out this work, we interviewed 234 people whose data were collected on a survey form for the occasion with patients of all ages (mothers answered on behalf of their children) at the laboratory to gather their informed opinions:

> Knowledge and attitudes about preventive measures to combat malaria > Causes of malaria transmission

> Regus care.

3.15 Management plan and data analysis

Data entry was ële done on Excel from the various registers (clinical and laboratory) and from the accompanying patient interview form. Data analysis was performed using SPSS software. Data analysis consisted of calculating :

- The annual incidence of malaria

- The frequency of signs/symptoms of malaria

- Frequency of use of GE and TDR

- Average parasitic load more or less ëstandard deviation

- The frequency of gamëtocyte carriage
- Frequency of use of malaria control measures

Frequency tables were used to present the qualitative variables. Means and standard deviations were calculated for the quantitative variables. The search for association between the qualitative variables was carried out using Chi2 statistical tests. Statistical inferences were made with an alpha risk of 0.05.

3.16 Quality control of thick drop reading :

A rapid and accurate biological diagnosis is necessary for the correct management of malaria. We drew 72 slides (positive and negative) read at the CSCOM during our routine visits for quality control by an experienced MRTC microscopist. It focused on the identification of plasmodial species and parasite counts. Sensitivity, specificity, kappa agreement and predictive values were calculated.

3.17 Ethical aspects :

We obtained authorisation from the Technical Director of the Mekin-Sikoro CSCOM, who explained the importance of the study to all his staff and the CSCOM management committee.

Ethical standards were respected throughout the interviewing of patients/carers by obtaining their verbal consent. There was no mention of the patient's name on the survey forms.

All the forms had identification codes that could not be traced back to the study participants.

It should be noted that all the patients agreed to cooperate with us without refusal, and others did not return after receiving the prescriptions for verification.

4 RESULTS

4.1 Analysis of registers (clinical and laboratory)

The study period from January to December 2021 enabled us to use the various registers of the CSCOM clinical consultation and laboratory.

In total, we analysed 6716 records of patients who had undergone thickened gout and/or RDT, of which 2140 (31.9%) were children aged 0 to 5 years.

4.1.1 Socio-demographic characteristics

The majority of the patients were women (58%), with a sex ratio of 1.38.

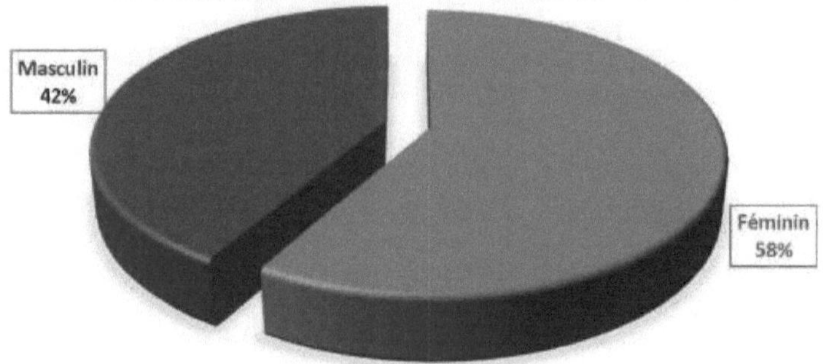

Figure 15: Breakdown of participants by gender

Table 7 ^Distribution of participants by age group

Age	Workforce	%
0-5 years	2140	31,9
6-10 years	642	9,6
11-20 years	1324	19,7
21-45 years old	2089	31,1
46-65 years old	383	5,7
> 65 years	138	2,1
Total	6716	100

The average age was 21.54 years, with a minimum of 1 month and a maximum of 85 years. The **0-5 age** group was in the majority in our study population with **31.9%**, followed by the **21-45 age** group with **31.1%**.

Ethnic group	Workforce	%
Bambara	2135	31,8
Dogon	589	8,8
Malinke	559	8,3
Peulh	805	12
Sarakole	1313	19,6
Senoufo	184	2,7
Sonrhai	318	4,7
Other	813	12,1

| Total | 6716 | 100 |

Other: Bozo; Kassonka; Wolof; Dafing; Mossi; Mianka; Maure; Bobo.

The Bambara ethnic group was in the majority, followed by the Sarakote, who represented 31.8% and 19.6% respectively.

Table 9: Rëpartition of patients by profession

Profession	Workforce	%
Retailer	**510**	**7,6**
Student	**1253**	**18,7**
Child	**1683**	**25,1**
Menagere	**1543**	**23**
Infant	**632**	**9,4**
Worker	**285**	**4,2**
Older people	**268**	**4**
Other	**542**	**8**
Total	**6716**	**100**

Other: Driver; Tailor; Electrician; Health worker; Teacher; Police officer.

Children and Mënagëres ëtaient les plus reprësentës dans notre ëtude soit respectivement 25,1% et 23% suivi des Eteves a 18,7%.

Table 10: Breakdown of patients by origin

Residence	Workforce	%
Banconi	**263**	**3,9**
Dialakorodji	**60**	**0,9**
Gabacoro	**105**	**1,6**
Gomi	**103**	**1,5**
Racecourse	**1125**	**16,8**
Sikoro	**4842**	**72,1**
Other	**218**	**3,2**
Total	**6716**	**100**

Others: Boulkassoumbougou ; Djëlibougou ; Mëdina-Coura, Nafadji ; Moribabougou ;
The majority of patients seen at the centre came from Sikoro, around 72.1%.

4.1.2 Clinical characteristics of patients :

Table 11: Breakdown of patients by reason for consultation during transmission periods (hot dry; cold dry; rainy season)

Symptoms/Month	N	Fever		Cephalees		Chills		Vomiting	
		n	%	n	%	N	%	n	%
				Hot dry season					
March	620	403	65	233	37,6	47	7,6	139	22,4
April	491	300	61,1	167	34	25	5,1	91	18,5
May	276	177	64,1	92	33,3	18	6,5	45	16,3
June	469	280	59,7	180	38,9	36	7,7	102	21,7

Total	**1856**	**1160**	**62,5**	**672**	**36,2**	**126**	**6,79**	**377**	**20,31**
			Cold season						
January	420	235	55,9	143	34,1	28	6,7	87	20,7
Fëvrier	348	183	52,6	122	35,1	16	4,6	55	15,8
November	530	394	74,3	268	50,6	88	16,6	131	24,7
Dëcembre	708	482	68,1	277	39,1	118	16,7	*201*	*28,4*
Total	**2006**	**1294**	**64,51**	**810**	**40,4**	**250**	**12,46**	**474**	**23,63**
			Rainy season						
July	586	393	67,1	236	40,3	76	13	115	19,6
August	771	488	63,3	273	35,4	99	12,8	194	25,2
September	688	413	60	286	41,6	81	11,8	133	19,3
October	809	526	65	435	53,8	126	15,6	203	25,1
Total	**2854**	**1820**	**63,77**	**1230**	**43,1**	**382**	**13,38**	**645**	**22,6**

Other: Courbature, abdominal pain, dizziness, diarrhoea, cough/cold, anorexia, weight loss

The most common signs in patients were fever (**64.51%**) in the cold season, followed by headache (**43.10%**) in the winter, vomiting (**23.63%**) in the cold season and shivering (**13.38%**) in the rainy season.

Table 12: Rëpartition of fever cases by age group.

Age/Death	Fever +	%	Total
0 to 5 years	1752	82	2140
6 to 15 years	808	70	1148
16 and over	1714	50	3425
Total	4274	64	6713

In our study, 82% of children under 5 years of age were most affected by fever. There was a statistically significant difference between age groups in the occurrence of fever (Chi^2 =- 603.7; OR=6.4; p< 10-3).

Table 13: Monthly breakdown of patients by sex.

Month		Male			Female		Total
	n	%	n			%	
January	158	37,62	262	62,38			420
February	139	39,94	209	60,06			348
March	249	40,16	371	59,84			620
April	176	35,85	315	64,15			491
May	115	41,67	161	58,33			276
June	179	38,17	290	61,83			469
July	241	41,13	345	58,87			586
August	333	43,19	438	56,81			771
September	320	46,51	368	53,49			688
October	372	45,98	437	54,02			809
November	216	40,75	314	59,25			530
December	299	42,23	409	57,77			708

| Total | 2797 | 41,65 | 3919 | 58,35 | 6716 |

Of the 6716 cases with a confirmatory malaria test, (3919) ëwere female (58%) and (2797) were male (42%). There was a statistically significant difference between the sexes during the months of the study (Chi^2 = 27, $p=0.005$).

4.1.3 Diagnostic profile of malaria

Table 14: Rëpartition of patients according to ëpaisse gout and RDT result (Laboratory Register).

Examination			Examination results		
	Positive	**%**	**Negative**	**%**	**Workforce**
GE	3435	51,5	3239	48,5	6674
TDR	15	18,75	65	81,25	80
Total	3450	0,51	3304	0,49	6754

From this distribution, we note that, 51.5% of participants had a positive ëpaisse gout as against 48.5% of negative ëpaisses gout.

Out of a total of 80 cases that benefited from RDT, 18.75% returned positive results.

Table 15: Distribution of patients according to seasons of transmission and ëpaisse gout result.

Month/GE	GE +	%	Total
	Dry season		
March	254	41,2	617
April	195	39,8	490
May	123	44,6	276
June	223	47,9	466
Total	795	43	1849
	Cold season		
January	160	38,7	413
February	146	42,6	343
November	355	67,6	525
December	327	46,3	706
Total	988	49,72	1987
	Rainy season		
July	317	54,5	582
August	389	51	763
September	386	56,4	685
October	560	69,3	808
Total	1652	58,21	2838

The rainy season (the months with high transmission) presented the highest number of positive thick drops in our study, around **58.21%** of cases; there was a statistically significant difference between the month and the thick drop result (Chi^2 =272.3, $p < 10$)$^{-3}$

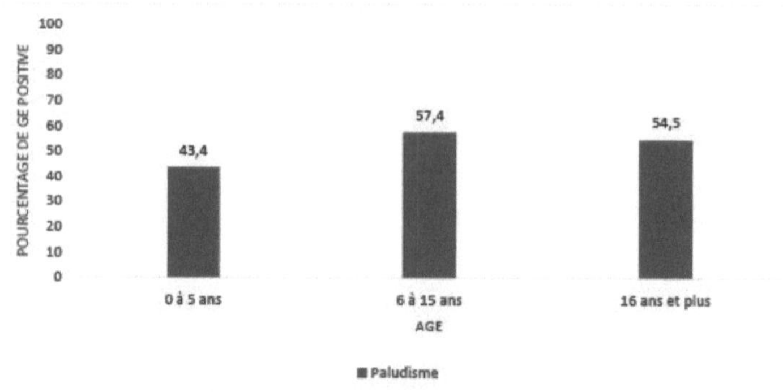

Figure 16: Rëpartition of malaria cases by age group.

The 6 to 15 age group had more positive ëpaisse gout during our, done there was a statistically significant difference between the age groups regarding thick gout ((Chi^2 = 84>5.99 ;p< 10^{-3} ; OR=2.5)

Tableau 16: Breakdown of patients by type of malaria (GE and/or RDT)

Malaria phenotype	Workforce	(%)
Simple malaria	3424	99,45
Severe malaria	19	0,55
Total	3435	100,00

Simple malaria was the most frequent, accounting for 99.45% of cases in our study.

4.1.4 Management of malaria cases :

Tableau 17: Rëpartition of patients according to antimalarial drugs regus and according to ëpaisse gout result.

Medication	Result of the thickened drop				Total
	Negative	%	Positive	%	N
Quinimax injection	398	20,65	1529	79,35	1927
Artesunate injection	125	17,46	577	80,59	702
Artemether injection	584	36,39	1021	63,61	1605
Amodiaquine syrup	282	95,92	12	4,08	294
Artemether-Lumefantrine cp	973	84,76	175	15,24	1148
Quinimax+ Artesunate injection	0	0	2	100	2
Quinimax+ Artemether injection	8	24,24	25	75,76	33
Quinimax+Arthemether-Lumefantrine cp	7	23,33	23	76,67	30
Artesunate+ Amodiaquine sp	0	0	4	100	4
Artesunate+ Artemether-Lumefantrine cp	0	0	6	100	6
Artemether injection+ Artemether-Lumefantrine cp	14	33,33	28	66,67	42
Sulfadoxine-pyrimethamine	1	100	0	00	1
Total	2392	41,18	3402	58,57	5794

In our ëtude we foundë that injectable quinine followed by ΓArtëmëther injectable and Art^sunate injectable ët were the anti-malarial drugs most present **73.1%** (4234/5794).

Tableau 18: Rëpartitions of patients according to treatment in severe malaria.

Medicines	Severe malaria		
	Workforce		(%)
Quinine	**injection9**		**47,37**
Artesunate	injection5		26,32
Artemether	injection1		5,26
Quinimax+	Artesunate1		5,26
Refere au CSRef	C13		15,79
Total19			**100**

In the management of severe malaria in our study, more than half of the cases were treated with injectable quinine (47.37%), followed by injectable artesunate (26.32%).

Table 19: Frequency of prescription of medicines associated with antimalarial treatment

Medicines	Numbers (N=6716)	(%)
Analgesics/Antipyretics	5698	84,8
Antibiotics	**6195**	**92,2**
Other medicines	4848	72,2

Other: vitamin B complex; iron + folic acid; dexamethasone; albendazole, etc.

Antibiotics (**92.2%**) and antipyretics (**84.8%**) were the drugs most frequently associated with antimalarial treatment.

Table 20: Rëpartition of patients by month and treatment compliance.

Seasons of Transmission/Processing	Compliant	%	Total
Hot dry season			
March	139	26,5	525
April	114	27,1	421
May	53	22,8	232
June	103	24,3	423
Total	**409**	**25,55**	**1601**
Cold season			
January	97	26,7	363
February	78	29,7	263
November	55	11,4	484
December	140	23,6	594
Total	**370**	**21,71**	**1704**
Rainy season			
July	97	18,7	519
August	141	21,6	654
September	114	18,8	606
October	107	14,1	757
Total	**459**	**18,1**	**2536**

Of the 5841 patients who received treatment for malaria, around 1238 people (21%) complied with the protocol laid down by the NMCP, so there was a statistically significant difference in treatment compliance depending on the month ($Chi^2 = 95, p< 10$).[-3]

Table 21: Rëpartition of patients according to compliance of antimalarial treatment with NMCP guidelines.

Treatment	Workforce	%
Compliant	**1238**	**21,2**
Non-compliant	4603	78,8
Total	**5841**	**100**

In 21.2% of cases, management was in line with the national treatment plan drawn up by the NMCP.

4.1.5 Quality control of the reading of thick drop slides

Table 22: Distribution of patients according to the result of the thick gout test at the MRTC - Parasitology and at the CSCOM of Sikoro

GE result		Result GE MRTC		Total
		Positive	Negative	
CSCOM Sikoro	Positive	24	29	53
	Negative	1	18	19
	Total	25	47	72

The sensitivity of the thickened drop reading was 96% in our study (24/25), a specificity of 38.3% (18/47), a positive predictive value of 45.3% (24/53) and a negative predictive value of 94.7% (18/19). Agreement between the two readings (CSCOM Sikoro versus MRTC - Parasitology) was **27.2%**.

4.2 Interviewing patients/parents : Use of malaria prevention measures

The study period from June 2022 to July 2023 enabled us to collect data from 234 people of all ages. All the people included had been diagnosed with malaria and treated at the Mekin-Sikoro CSCom.

Table 23: Ways of preventing malaria

Means of prevention	Yes		No		Often		Total
	Workforce	%	Workforce	%	Workforce	%	
ITN use	157	66,5	77	32,6	2	0,9	236
SP/FE socket	5	31,3	11	68,7	0	0	16

The majority of people surveyed (66.5%) in our study used insecticide-treated mosquito nets to prevent malaria.

More than half **(68.7%)** of the pregnant women surveyed had not taken at least one dose of Sulfadoxine-pyrimethamine prior to the survey.

Tableau 24: Knowledge of the cause of malaria transmission by patients/parents

Causes	Workforce	%
Mosquito	**183**	**77,5**
Other	**47**	**19,9**
Mosquito and Other	**6**	**2,5**
Total	**236**	**100**

77.5% of people surveyed knew that malaria is transmitted by mosquitoes.

Tableau 25: Rëpartition of patients interviewedës according to 1 biological examination ийНзё for confirmation of malaria diagnosis.

Examination	Workforce	%
GE	**201**	**85,2**
TDR	4	1,7
GE and TDR	31	13,1
Total	**236**	**100**

Of the patients with Ьёпёййё a biological test to confirm the diagnosis, **85.2%** ëtaited ëpaisse gout versus **1.7%** TDR.

Tableau 26: Rate of positive gout ëpaisse (GE) in Interviewës patients.

Result	Workforce	%
Positive	**82**	**34,7**
№gative	154	65,3
Total	**236**	**100**

In our survey, we noted that, **65.3%** of participants had iregative ëpaisse gout versus **34.7%** who had positive ëpaisse gout.

5 Comment and Discussion :

The results obtained from the mëthodology we applied prompted comment and discussion in relation to the results of other similar studies.

- SOCIO-DEMOGRAPHIC CHARACTERISTICS :

> **Age**

The average age was 21.54 years, with a minimum of 1 month and a maximum of 85 years.

Our study showed that the **0-5** age group was the most represented, with 2,140 people **(31.9%)**, followed by the **21-45 age** group **(31.1%)**. This result is similar to that of **Sidibe. I in 2019 in commune III of the district of Bamako**, who found 43.27% [**67**], which seems to be linked to the fact that this age group is the most vulnerable because it has no premunition.

> **Gender**

In total, we recorded 6716 participants during our survey at the Mekin-Sikoro CSCom, with a sex ratio in favour of women of 1.38, i.e. **58%.** This result is consistent with that found by **Fomba.S et *al* in 2018** during their study in commune V of the Bamako district [**64**], who found a female predominance of 57.3%. In contrast, **Oureiba.A** in Kalifabougou in 2021 [**2**] found **51.6%** gargons and **48.4%** girls, with a sex ratio of 1.06 in favour of males.

This difference could be explained by the frequency of women in households at the time of data collection in our study.

> **Ethnic group**

In our study population the Bambara ethnic group was the most represented with **31.8%** followed by Sarakole which represented **19.6%.** The result of our study was inferior to that of **Dia.S** et *al* in Kambila (Kati) in 2011[**23**] who found that Bambara was more represented with **59.56%** of the total population followed by Sarakoles **(34.22%)**, Peulhs **(4.89%)** and Malinkes **(1.33%).** This difference could be explained by the zonal distribution of ethnic groups in Mali.

> **Residence**

In terms of the health area, the majority of malaria cases reported resided in Mёкт- Sikoro with a prevalence of **72.1%,** which is an important element in Mali's health policy of bringing care closer to the population.

> **Profession or Occupation**

Children not attending school and menagëres were the most represented with respectively 25.1% and 23%, followed by pupils at 18.7%. These figures are comparable to those obtained by **Kone.C et *al.* in Bancoumana in 2020 (Kati) [65]**; who found 29.3% and 26.0% respectively among children and menagëers, followed by pupils and farmers.

• **The main clinical manifestations encountered during the study period** :

The diagnosis of presumptive malaria, made after clinical examination, was most often based on clinical signs suggestive of malaria. The main signs reported by patients in our study were fever (63.6%), followed by headache (40.44%), cough/cold (28.8%) and vomiting (22.3%); similar results were observed in the **Dia.S et al. in Kambila (Kati) in 2011[23)]**, in which fever was the most common sign among malaria cases (41.46%), followed by headache (36.16%), abdominal pain (13.76%) and vomiting (9.61%);

This could be explained by the fact that people are much more familiar with the first steps to take in the event of fever in children.

The month of October was the most represented, with 17.8% of cases, corresponding to the peak of high seasonal transmission.

- **Diagnostic profile :**

Our results showed that the most commonly used diagnostic test was the thick drop with 85.1% of patients interviewed, in line with that of **Guindo.D** in **Kalabancoro in 2020** who found 78% of cases of thick drop in his study **[66]**. This may be justified by the fact that it is recommended by the malaria management guidelines concerning diagnosis. These guidelines stipulate that when malaria is suspected, it is imperative to carry out a diagnostic test (RDT, thick drop). It should also be added that the cost is accessible to the population; it was available at the ASACOMSI during our study. We should also add that it is more spëcific than the RDT, which cannot give parasitaemia.

With only 18.75% of diagnoses confirmed by an RDT, our result is similar to that of the 2018 Mali Demographic and Health Surveys with 19% of positive RDTs in children under 5 years of age **[5]**. Unlike that of **OUREIBA.A in Kalifabougou in 2021[2], the** prevalence of malaria confirmed by RDT was 97.8% in his study. This difference could be explained by the fact that RDTs were not used systematically for the biological confirmation of malaria at the Mekin-Sikoro community health centre.

- **Therapeutic profile :**

The survey of therapeutic itineraries showed that :

Quinine and Artemether were the most prescribed antimalarial drugs, respectively 44.95% and 30.01%, followed by Artesunate 16.96%.

Antimalarial treatment administered during our study complied with national guidelines in 21.2% of cases, in contrast to the result obtained by **Sidibe. I in 2019 in commune III of the Bamako district**, who found that 90.97% of drug prescriptions complied with those recommended by the PNLP **[67]**. The inadequacy of the treatment often concerned both the choice of molecule and the dosage.

This could be explained by the fact that the cost of quinine could influence prescribers' motivation to prescribe it.

This non-compliance could also be due to inadequate training of healthcare staff in malaria management, in line with the NMCP's policy framework.

Knowledge of how malaria is transmitted

In our study, mosquito bites were most frequently mentioned by 77.5% of participants. This rate could possibly be explained by the impact of awareness-raising and mass distribution of ITNs in the Bamako health district. This result is close to those obtained by the **Enquete sur les Indicateurs du Paludisme (EIPM) in 2021 [71]** and by the **EDSM-VI in 2018 [5]**, respectively 72.7% and 73%; it is clearly higher than those obtained by **C. NDO et al in September 2011 in Cameroon [72]**, who found 69%. These results could be explained in part by greater acceptance by the population of the benefits of using ITNs, but also by the ever-increasing efforts of the NMCP and its partners to provide the population with means of preventing malaria infection.

Most of the participants (77.5%) cited the bite of the female anopheles as the mode of transmission of malaria, while others cited: the consumption of eggs, the consumption of fruit and/or vegetables that were not washed or were poorly washed, the consumption of foods rich in fat, the consumption of unfit food and the consumption of dirty water. This result is similar to that obtained by **C. NDO et al in September 2011 in Cameroon [72]**, who found mosquito bites to be 82% of the cause of malaria in their study.

- **Means of combating malaria**

In our study, the majority of people knew the means of preventing malaria. Among them, the insecticide-impregnated mosquito net was the method most known and used by the population with 66.5% compared to other methods, which is clearly lower than that obtained by **Larissa TAGNE MEKOWA. L** in Koulouba, Sogonafing and Point G in 2021 found 85.55% **[68].** This difference can be explained by the fact that our subjects used other means of protection against malaria apart from the mosquito net, and also that not all of them had a mosquito net.

More than half **(68.7%)** of the pregnant women surveyed stated that they had not taken at least one dose of Sulfadoxine-pyrimethamine prior to the survey. This can be explained by the fact that the survey was carried out at the laboratory during their first prenatal check-up, i.e. the first trimester of pregnancy.

Quality control

Since March 2009, the WHO (WHO, PNLP-MALI 2016) **[61] has** recommended a biological diagnosis prior to any anti-malarial treatment. A rapid and accurate biological diagnosis is necessary for the correct management of malaria. Thus, for quality control, a total of 72 slides were taken at random from the CSCOM of Mekin-Sikoro. The quality control results showed agreement with kappa (27.2%), good sensitivity (96%), poor specificity (38.7%) and predictive values (positive predictive value: 45.3%; acceptable negative predictive value: 94.7%).

Only the *Plasmodium falciparum* species was diagnosed at Mekin-Sikoro and the MRTC for quality control Quality control of the reading of thick ë drops during a тепёе study at different levels of the health pyramid in Mali indicated 56% false positive results and a concordance of 49,3% compared with the results of the reference service, the Departement d'Epidemiologie des Affections Parasitaires (DEAP) according to a study conducted by **A. Dolo et al in 2010 [73].** The causes of discrepancies were purely quantitative.

Limitations of the study :

Although our study has produced results that may be useful for policy, it does have some limitations that should be taken into account:

- Under-application of biological diagnostic tools (RDTs) ;
- The failure to systematically report all the clinical and biological data on malaria in the consultation register.
- There was little information in the literature review on the proper management of malaria in the study area, which raised some questions during the discussion.
- Disregarding CPS, fumigation and intra-domiciliary spraying as preventive measures

6 CONCLUSION

Malaria 6was the most frequent cause of consultation at the CSCOM of Mёкт-Sikoro. This frequency is Hёc a seasonal^ of malaria with the maximum number of cases in pёriode hivernale (July-October) with a great susceptibility^ of cases in children aged 6-15 years. The most frequent clinical signs were fever, headache, vomiting and chills. Good knowledge of how to prevent malaria
Efforts needed to improve adherence to the national malaria management policy

7 RECOMMENDATIONS

In the light of these results on the management of malaria, we make the following recommendations, addressed respectively to :

-       **The health authorities (Ministry of Health, PNLP, Direction Générale de la Santé, etc.).**

Health)

- Providing training/refresher courses for staff on malaria management (diagnosis, clinic and treatment).

- Health service providers:

- Raise public awareness of the need to sleep under insecticide-impregnated mosquito nets;
- Adhere to and apply the directives of the national malaria control policy

- To the public

- Getting children into health centres early.
- Cleaning up living spaces.
- Sleep under a mosquito net.
- Focus on malaria prevention, especially for children under 5 and pregnant women.

> Carrying out a thick drop versus rapid diagnostic test (RDT) study

> Quality control of thick drops read at the CSCOM at MRTC level

BIBLIOGRAPHICAL REFERENCES :

1. **Robert V, Chippaux JP, Diomande L.** Le Paludisme en Afrique de 1 1 Ouest : ëtudes entomologiques et ëpidëmiologiques en zone rizicole et en milieu urbain. IRD Editions; 1991

2. **Oureiba A.** Evaluation du paludisme chez les enfants de 0 a 5 ans au CSCom de Kalifabougou (Kati). USTTB; These Med 2021

3. **World Malaria Report 2022**: new tools are needed to reach global malaria targets | Target Malaria. [Cite 12 Feb. 2023].

4. **Local Health Information System - SLIS.** [Cite 12 fevr. 2023].

5. **Institut National de la Statistique (INSTAT).** Enquete Demographique et de Sante 2018 EDSM_VI. Bamako, Mali: Institut National de la Statistique (INSTAT) Bamako, Mali; 2019

6. **Greenwood BM, Fidock DA, Kyle DE, Kappe SHI, Alonso PL, Collins FH, et al.** Review series Malaria: progress, perils, and prospects for eradication. J Clin Invest. 2008 [cite 15 feb. 2023] ;118(4) :1266-76. Available at: http://www.jci.org

7. **World-malaria-report-2020-briefing-kit-fre.**

8. **Africa memoir**: Generalities About Malaria. [Cited 16 Feb. 2023]. Available at: https://www.africmemoire.com

9. **AMOUSSOUVI.AAL** Etude comparative des résultats de la goutte épaisse faite a partir du sang capillaire et celle confectionnee sur du sang veineux au Centre Medical Saint Jean de Cotonou. [Bëɯɯ] : UNIVERSITE D'ABOMEY-CALAVI ; EPAC/UAC ; [Cite 16 fevr. 2023]. These Med 2018

10. **Rema.R** Etude des perturbations hematologiques observeses au cours de la crise aigue du paludisme chez 1 enfant au service de pëdiatrie du Centre Hospitalier National Yalgado Ouedraogo (CHN-YO). 1998 ;

11. **Cox FE**. History of the discovery of the malaria parasites and their vectors. Parasit Vectors. 2010 [cite 25 feb. 2023] ;3(1) :5.
Available at: /pmc/articles/PMC2825508/

12. **World Malaria Day**: WHO launches efforts to eradicate malaria in an additional 25 countries by 2025. [Cite 17 Feb 2023].
Available at : https://www.who.int/fr

13. **Pierre Aubry, Bernard-Alex Gauzere.** Malaria.pdf. [Cite 26 March 2022]. Available at: http://medecinetropicale.free.fr/cours/paludisme.pdf

14. **Rogier C HMJF. Rogier C et al** Evaluation epidemiologique du paludisme en zone d'endëmie. Mëdecine Tropicale [Internet]. 2009 [cite 8 mars 2023] ;2(69) :123-42

15. **Doumbo O.** Epidëmiologie du paludisme au Mali: etude de la chloroquinoresistance, essai de stratëgie de controle basee sur l'utilisation de rideaux impregnes de permethrine associee au traitement systëmatique des acces fëbriles. http://www.theses.fr .1janv.1992[cite 17 fëvr. 2023] ; Available from: http://www.theses.fr/1992

16. **ANOFEL**, malaria. 2021 - Google search [Internet]. [Cite 5 Feb. 2023]. Available at: https://www.google.com

17. **Deschamps S.** Etude de la diversite et de la crucialite des voies de synthese des phospholipides structuraux chez differentes especes de Plasmodium.1janv.2009 [cite 18 fevr. 2023] ; Available at: http://www.theses.fr/2009MON20260

18. **Rich SM, Leendertz FH, Xu G, LeBreton M, Djoko CF, Aminake MN, et al. The** Origin of malignant malaria. Proc Natl Acad Sci USA. 1 Sep 2009 [cite 18 Feb 2023]

;106(35) :14902-7.Available at: https://pubmed.ncbi.nlm.nih.gov

19. **Malaria (ANOFEL)** Association Frangaise des Enseignants de Parasitologie et Mycologie 2014. [Cite 17 Feb 2023]. Available at: https://fr.readkong.com

20. **Culleton R, Coban C, Zeyrek FY, Cravo P, Kaneko A, Randrianarivelojosia M, et al.** The Origins of African. *Plasmodium vivax*; insights from mitochondrial genome sequencing. PLoS One [Internet]. 14 Dec 2011 [cite 18 Feb 2023] ;6(12).

Available at : https://pubmed.ncbi.nlm.nih.gov

21. **Howes RE, Battle KE, Mendis KN, Smith DL, Cibulskis RE, Baird JK, et al.** Global Epidemiology of Plasmodium vivax. Am J Trop Med Hyg. 2016 [cite 18 Feb. 2023] ;95(6 Suppl.) :15-34. Available at: https://pubmed.ncbi.nlm.nih.gov

22. **Amele Nyedzie WOTODJO.** Study of malaria in adults in two villages in Senegal: Dielmo and Ndiop. [Cite 19 fevr 2023].

23. **Dia.S**, Epidemiology of malaria in a Sudano-Guinean area of Mali, Kambila cercle de Kati. Universite de Bamako, Faculte de Medecine, de Pharmacie et d'Odonto- Stomatologie. These Med 2011, 22p. [cite 1 fevr 2023] ;

24. **Kei'ta M. Baber N. Sogoba M. Maiga B. Diallo S.et al** (2014) Vector-borne malaria transmission in a village on the banks of the River Niger and its fishing hamlet (Kenieroba and Fourda, Mali). December, Volume 107, Issue 5, pp 356-368

25. **Diallo M, Sangare D, Diarra A, Camara D, Mariko R, Guidenarhd M, et al**. Study of the adult population dynamics *of Anopheles gambiae s.l.* and the allelic polymorphism of the TEP1 gene during malaria transmission in the rural commune of Bancoumana, Mali. Rev Mali Infect Microbiol. 1 Apr 2017 [cite 19 Feb 2023] ;9(1) :48-55.

Available at : https://doaj.org

26. **Sylla. D**: Trophic behaviour of Anopheles gambiae and other mosquito species for different hosts in Selingue, Mali. [Mali]: FMOS; 2015 [сЛё 12 March 2023]. Available from: https://www.bibliosante.ml

27. **WHO.** Malaria. Available at   https://www.who.int/fr/news-room/fact-sheets/detail/malaria. Accessed 25 Feb. 2023.2021 Report

28. **Robert V, Boudin C.** Biology of human-mosquito transmission of plasmodium. Parasitology. Manuscript n°2454a. 2002

29. **Kean BH, Reilly PC.** Malaria - the mime. Recent lessons from a group of civilian travellers. Am J Med. 1976 [cite 25 feb 2023] ;61(2) :159-64.

Available at: https://pubmed.ncbi.nlm.nih.gov/782238/

30. **Madamet M.T.** Influence of environmental conditions on the metabolism of Plasmodium falciparum. Institut de Medecine Tropicale du service de sante des Armees. IRBA Antenne de Marseille. 2010 -. [Cite 1 mars 2023].

31. **Eichner M, Diebner HH, Molineaux L, Collins WE, Jeffery GM, Dietz K.** Genesis, sequestration and survival of Plasmodium falciparum gametocytes: parameter estimates from fitting a model to malariatherapy data. Trans R Soc Trop Med Hyg. 2001 [cite 1 mars 2023] ;95(5) :497-501.

Available at: https://pubmed.ncbi.nlm.nih.gov/11706658/

32. **Plasmodium life cycle** - Professional edition of the MSD Manual. [Cite 25 fevr.2023]. Available at: https://www.merckmanuals.com/fr-ca/professional/multimedia/figure/cycle-de-vie-de-plasmodium

33. **Cranston HA**, Boylan CW, Carroll GL, Sutera SP, Williamson JR, Gluzman IY, et al. Plasmodium falciparum Maturation Abolishes Physiologic Red Cell Deformability. Science

(1979). [Cite 12 March 2023] ;223(4634) :400-3.

Available at: https://www.science.org/doi/10.1126/science.6362007

34. **AMBROISE THOMAS P., CARNEVALE P., FELIX H., MOUCHET J**. Malaria Encycl. Med. Chir (Paris), Maladies infectieuses 8089, 1984; p10 and p 20. [Cite 26 fevr 2023] Available at : https://pubmed.ncbi.nlm.nih.gov/1327352/

35. Association Frangaise des Enseignants de Parasitologie et Mycologie R ANOFEL ; 31 Aout ; 2008cour parasitologie ; 31Aout 2008

36. Association Frangaise des Enseignants de Parasitologie et Mycologie ANOFEL. Parasitology course 2014

http://campus.cerimes.fr/parasitologie/polyparasitologie.pdf ; 411(77) :21-24 ; [cite 10 mars 2023].

37. **Diawara AA.** Epidëmiologie clinique du paludisme grave chez les enfants de 06-59 mois a Bamako, Bandiagara et a Sikasso dans un contexte de mise a 6chelle des stratëgies de lutte.. [BAMAKO]: FMOS; 2019 [екё 10 March 2023].

Available at : https://www.bibliosante.ml/handle/123456789/3677

38. **MARLENE ALVINE P.** Etude bibliographique des theses rëalisëes sur le paludisme a la FMPOS, de janvier 2007 a dëcembre 2008 -. [Bamako]: FMPOS; [екё 12 March 2023].

39. **WHO**. Module de formation a la lutte antipaludique: prise en charge du paludisme. 2014 [cË1ё 26 March 2023];

Available   at:

https://apps.who.mt/iris/bitstreamr/handle/10665/112845/9789242503975_fre.pdf

40. **MP Brenier-Pinchart, Pinel C, Grillot R, Ambroise-Thomas P.** Le diagnostic du paludisme dans les régions non endëmiques : valeur, limites et complëmentaritë des mëthodes actuelles. anofel.net. 2000 [ci^ 16 march 2023] ;3(58) :310-6

41. **Dejazmach Z, Alemu G, Yimer M, Tegegne B, Getaneh A**. Assessing the Performance of CareStart[TM] Malaria Rapid Diagnostic Tests in Northwest Ethiopia: A Cross-Sectional Study. 2021 [екё 17 March 2023] ;

Available at: https://doi.org/10.1155/2021/7919984

42. **Incardona S, Serra-Casas E, Champouillon N, Nsanzabana C, Cunningham J, Gonzalez IJ.** Global survey of malaria rapid diagnostic test (RDT) sales, procurement and lot verification practices: assessing the use of the WHO-FIND Malaria RDT Evaluation Programme (20112014). Malar J [Internet]. 15 May 2017 [^1ё 17 March 2023] ;16(1):196. Available at: /pmc/articles/PMC543307 8/

43. **Colin L, Mallie M, Bastide JM.** Rapid diagnosis of malaria by testing for circulating antigënes. Revue Frangaise des Laboratoires. 1 jan. 2000 ;2000(319) :59-64.

44. **M.P. Brenier-Pinchart, C. Pinel, R. Grillot, P. Ambroise-Thomas**. Diagnosis of malaria in non-endëmic regions: value, limitations, and complëmentaritë of current mëthods. Ann Biol Clin. 5 Jan. 2000 [^Tё 23 Apr. 2023] ;58 :310-5.

Available at : https://anofel.net/images/accreditation/bibliographie/palu abc.pdf

45. **CAVALLO JD, HERNANDEZ E, GEROME P, PLOITON N, DEBORD T, LE VAGUERESSE R.** Antigënëmie HRP-2 and imported Plasmodium falciparum malaria: Comparison of ParaSight-F® and ICT malaria P.®. Mëdecine tropicale. 1997 ;57(4) :353-6.

46. **Grobusch MP, Alpermann U, Schwenke S, Jelinek T, Warhurst DC.** False-positive rapid tests for malaria in patients with rheumatoid factor. Lancet. 23 Jan 1999 [cite 23 Apr 2023];353(9149):297. Available at : http://www.thelancet.com

47. **Lee N, Baker J, Andrews KT, Gatton ML, Bell D, Cheng Q, et al.** Effect of sequence variation in Plasmodium falciparum histidine-rich protein 2 on binding of specific monoclonal antibodies: Implications for rapid diagnostic tests for malaria. J Clin Microbiol. Aug 2006 [cite 23 Apr 2023] ;44(8) :2773-8.
Available at: https://journals.asm.org/doi/10.1128/JCM.02557-05

48. **Hance P, Garnotel E, De Pina JJ, Vedy S, Ragot C, Chadli M, et al.** Rapid immunochromatographic tests for malaria detection, principles and strategies of use. Med Trop. 2005 ;65 :389-93

49. **Minodier P.** Depistage du paludisme : tests rapides.J Pediatr Pueric.1 dec 2005;18(8) :386-8.

50. **Grobusch MP, Hanscheid T, Zoller T, Jelinek T, Burchard GD.** Rapid immunochromatographic malarial antigen detection unreliable for detecting Plasmodium malariae and Plasmodium ovale. European Journal of Clinical Microbiology and Infectious Diseases. 2002 [cite 24 Apr 2023] ;21(11) :818-20.

51. **Rogier C, Henry M, tropicale JTM, 2009.** Evaluation epidemiologique du paludisme en zone d'endëmie. horizon.documentation.ird.fr. 2009 [cite 24 Apr. 2023] ;62(2) : 123-42.

52. **WHO.** Guidelines for the treatment of malaria. 16 February 2021 [Internet]. 2021 [cited 2023 May 28]. p. 68

53. **TAPSOBA Serge Pascal.** Evaluation of the application of national guidelines for the diagnosis and treatment of malaria at the hospital centre. [Burkina Faso] ; these phar 2013 [cited 2023 May 28].

54. **Pr. E. Pichard Pr MD.** les-anti-paludiques.pdf. 2003

55. **Ako A.** Evolution of resistance to sulfadoxine-pyrimethamine and chloroquine, and analysis of the complexity of Plasmodium falciparum infections, Welch (1897) in. 2014 [cited 2023 Jun 9] ; https://hal.science/tel-02885141/

56. **Jaeger A, Sauder P, Kopferschmitt J, Flesch F.** Clinical features and management of poisoning due to antimalarial drugs. Med Toxicol Adverse Drug Exp. 1987 [cited 2023 Jun 8] ;2(4) :242-73. https://pubmed.ncbi.nlm.nih.gov/3306266/

57. **Winstanley P, Coleman J, Maggs J, Breckenridge A, Park B.** The toxicity of amodiaquine and its principal metabolites towards mononuclear leucocytes and granulocyte/monocyte colony forming units. Br J Clin Pharmacol. 1990 [cited 2023 Jun 9] ;29(4) :479-85. https://pubmed.ncbi.nlm.nih.gov/2328196

58. **Kloprogge F, McGready R, Hanpithakpong W, Blessborn D, Day NPJ, White NJ, et al.** Lumefantrine and Desbutyl-Lumefantrine Population Pharmacokinetic-Pharmacodynamic Relationships in Pregnant Women with Uncomplicated Plasmodium falciparum Malaria on the Thailand-Myanmar Border. Antimicrob Agents Chemother. 2015 Oct 1 [cited 2023 Jun 9] ;59(10) :6375-84. https://pubmed.ncbi.nlm.nih.gov/26239986/

59. **Sagara I, Beavogui AH, Zongo I, Soulama I, Borghini-Fuhrer I, Fofana B, et al.** Pyronaridine-artesunate or dihydroartemisinin-piperaquine versus current first-line therapies for repeated treatment of uncomplicated malaria: a randomised, multicentre, open-label, longitudinal, controlled, phase 3b/4 trial. Lancet. 2018 APR 7 [cited 2023 Jun 9] ;391(10128) :1378-90. https://pubmed.ncbi.nlm.nih.gov/29606364/

60. **Famanta A, Diakite M, Diawara SI, Diakite SA, Doumbia S, Traore K, et al.** Prevalence of maternal, placental and low birth weight malaria during labour and *postpartum* in përшгьат a Bamako (Mali). Cahiers d^tudes et de recherches francophones/Sante.20ll.lul 1 [cited 2023 Jun 9] ;21(1) :3-7. https://www.jle.com/fr

61. **Programme national de lutte contre le paludisme** p. directives nationales de prise en charge des cas de paludisme au Mali. Pnlp mali; 2020.

62. **Sundararaman SA, Odom John AR**. Prevention of malaria in pregnancy: The threat of sulfadoxine-pyrimethamine resistance. Front Pediatr. 18 August 2022;10.

63. **Chotsiri P, White NJ, Tarning J**. Pharmacokinetic considerations in seasonal malaria chemoprevention. Trends Parasitol. 1 August 2022 [cited 13 June 2023] ;38(8) :673-82. Available at : https://pubmed.ncbi.nlm.nih.gov/35688778/

64. **Eastman RT, Fidock DA, Richard T.** Artemisinin-based combination therapies: a vital tool in efforts to eliminate malaria.
Available at: http://www.gatesfoundation.org/Pages/home.aspx

66. **Fomba S**, Coulibaly C, Bamba, Toure F, Sangho H. Effet de la formation sur la qualité de la prise en charge des cas de paludisme dans les centres de sante de premier contact de la commune V de Bamako. Sciences de la Sante. 2018 [cited 28 Jul 2023] ;41(2). Available at: https://revuesciencestechniquesburkina.org/index.php/sciences_de_la_sante/article/view/691

67. **Kone C**. La Place du paludisme dans les consultations au centre de sante communautaire (CSCOM) de Bancoumana cercle de Kati, Mali. These Med 2020 [cite 29 Jul 2023]; Available at: https://www.bibliosante.ml/handle/123456789/3870

68. **Guindo.D** : Prise en charge du Paludisme chez les enfants de six a cinquante-neuf mois dans trois Cscom du district sanitaire de Kalabancoro 2020 . [Cite 31 Jul 2023]. These Med 2020 Available at : https://bibliosante.ml/handle/123456789/4181

69. **Sidibe I.** Etude de la conformite des prescriptions antipaludiques aux normes et directives du programme national de lutte contre le paludisme dans le centre de Sante de. These Phar 2019 [cite 3 aout 2023] ; Available at: https://bibliosante.ml/handle/123456789/4897

70. **Tagne Mekowa LL**. Paludisme : connaissances, pratiques de prévention et itineraries therapeutiques a Koulouba, Sogonafing et Point G (Bamako, mali). These Med 2021 [cited 3 Aug 2023]; Available at: https://www.bibliosante.ml/handle/123456789/4599

71. Institut National de la Statistique (INSTAT), Programme National de Lutte contre le Paludisme (PNLP) and ICF. 2021. Enquete sur les Indicateurs du Paludisme au Mali 2021 Available at: https://www.dhsprogram.com

72. **Ndo C, Menze-Djantio B, Antonio-Nkondjio C**. Awareness, attitudes and prevention of malaria in the cities of Douala and Yaounde (Cameroon). Parasit Vectors [Internet]. 20 Sep 2011];4(1):181. Available from: https://doi.org/10.1186/1756-3305-4-181

73. **Dolo A., Diallo M., Saye R., Konare A., Ouattara A., Poudiougo B., Kouyate B., Minta D., Doumbo OK.** (2010): "Problematique du diagnostic biologique du paludisme au Mali - Perspectives". Med Trop 2010; 70: 158-162.

APPENDICES

Malaria survey sheet CSCOM Mekin-Sikoro

(Interview with patient or patient's relative)

No. Lab register TDR)	Type of diagnosis (GE,	Result diagnostic	Malaria prevention	Treatment malaria	Cause of malaria
(1=GE, 2=TDR) 2=No)	SP Date used Start date (1=positive, if FE ? symptoms of care (1=Yes, Used 2=negative) (1=Yes,	DateM (1=Yes, treatment received 2=No)2=other	LLIN1=mosquito,		

Thick drop technique

Materials required: OMS slide collection box, new slides, vaccinostyl, 90° alcohol, Giemsa solution, cotton wool, binocular microscope, ratelier, timer, record book, polyvinyl gloves, hygienic steel, staining tray, buffer Tablet Ph = 7.2 (1 tablet per litre of water).

Procedure for thick gout

The EW was performed using blood taken from one of the fingers of the hand. The finger was disinfected with an alcohol swab. Using a single-use vaccinostyl, a capillary puncture was made on the pulp of the disinfected finger. The firstère drop a ёlё ёHттёe with dry cotton. The second drop dёposёe in the middle of a slide with the angle of a secondiёme slide, the dёfibrillation mёcanique a ёlё done by circular movements that started from the centre a la pёriphёrie of the slide so as to ёtaler blood in a circle of about 1 cm diamёtre. The slides were ёlё sёchёed at the tempёrature of the collection room away from dust, sunlight and flies. Slides were stained with 3% Giemsa stain diluted in buffer water at Ph = 7.2 for 30 minutes, then rinsed and dried.

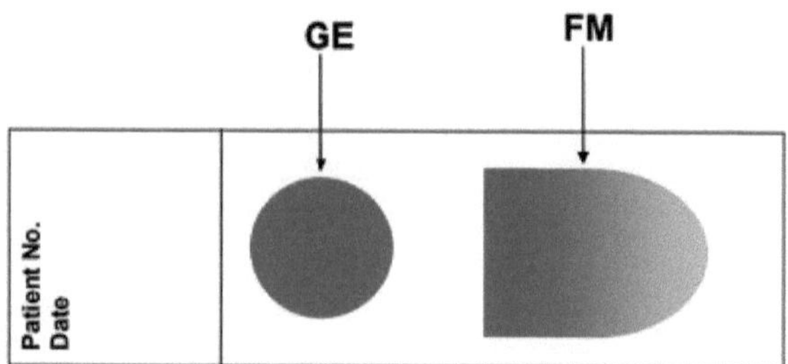

Figure 17: Fabrication of the GE and FM on a single object-holder blade

- Is not fixëe! The mëthanol used to fix the FM must not touch the GE
- Red blood cells are absent (Гузёз by water with staining)
- More sensitive than smears for determining the presence/absence of parasites
- иШ18ё to dëtermine parasite density in most cases.

Thin smear :

Making the thin smear

- The smear must be taken with care so as to ensure that only one layer is used. mobile phone.
- The colouring must not contain any deposits of dyes that would generate and could cause errors.
- A drop of blood is tested using a second slide as a spreader or a coverslip.
- Place the edge of the spreader 1cm in front of the single drop, move it closer until it touches the drop, leave to melt and spread.
- Remove Etaleur quickly to reveal a tail
- Spread the remaining 3 drops of blood in a circle about 1 cm in diameter using the corner of the spatula.
- The smear should not be too thick or too thin (you should be able to read the typewritten letters through the film).

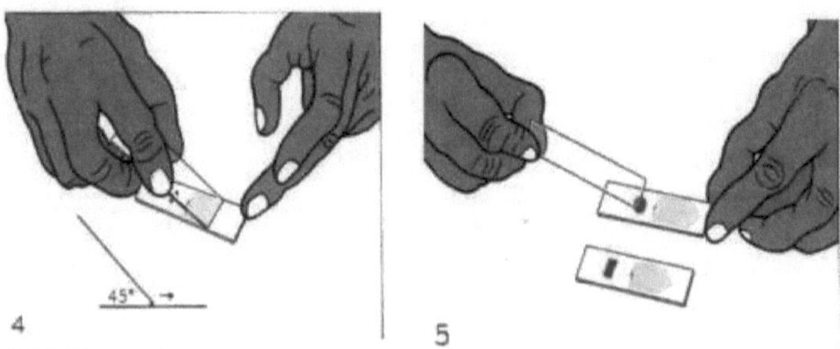

Figure 18: Making a thin smear

- A ëtaler first and 1cm away from the GE
- Fixë with absolute mëthanol
- Presence of a tail
- The red blood cells are intact and their morphology can be examined.
- Specifique to determine the morphology of the parasite

70

<u>Determination of parasitaemia according to the WHO calculation (2009)</u> :

Let's assume 8000 WBC (White Blood Cells) per microlitre:

8000 GB/pl = N parasites/pl

GB counts parasites counts N parasites/pl = 8000 x parasites counts/ GB counts **<u>Example</u>**: 87 parasites are counted for 504 GB N parasites/pl = (8000 x 87) /504 = ... Parasites/pl

<u>TDR operating procedure</u> :

a)   Bring the contents of the paracheck Pf® box to room temperature before testing in the open air (if stored in the refrigerator).

b)   Open the sachet and remove the cassette. Once the sachet has been opened, the cassette should be used immediately. But before use, check the colour of the desiccant. It should be blue. If it has become colourless or pale blue, discard it and use another. The plastic frame of the test should be marked with the patient's name or code, the date and the exact time (hour and minute).

c)   Clean the chosen area, either the finger (palmar surface of the tip of the 3rd or 4th left prëfërence finger), or the big toe or heel in infants, with an alcohol-soaked cotton pad. Then leave it to dry for a few seconds (or clean with dry swab) with the left hand press firmly on the proximal part of the cleaned finger to stimulate circulation and using a sterile vaccinostyle.

d)   Prick the chosen area with one controlled movement. With one hand, squeeze the finger to draw a drop of blood. With the other hand, hold the pipette in the middle and bring the pipette into contact with the surface of the drop of blood: the right amount of blood (about 5pl) will be collected by the action of surface tension.

e)   Transfer the blood thus collected onto the test pad, into sampling port A a whole blood sample of 5pl can thus be obtained or a micro-pipette can also be used to transfer 5pl of the anti-clotting or finger prick sample onto the test pad, into sampling port A.

f)   Homogenise the anticoagulant blood sample by gentle mixing. Bring the sample loop into contact with the surface of the blood sample contained in the container, ensuring that the blood from the sample loop will be fully absorbed by the test buffer. Place 6 drops (300pl) of wash buffer into sample port B', holding the plastic dropper firmly. After 15 minutes, read the results.

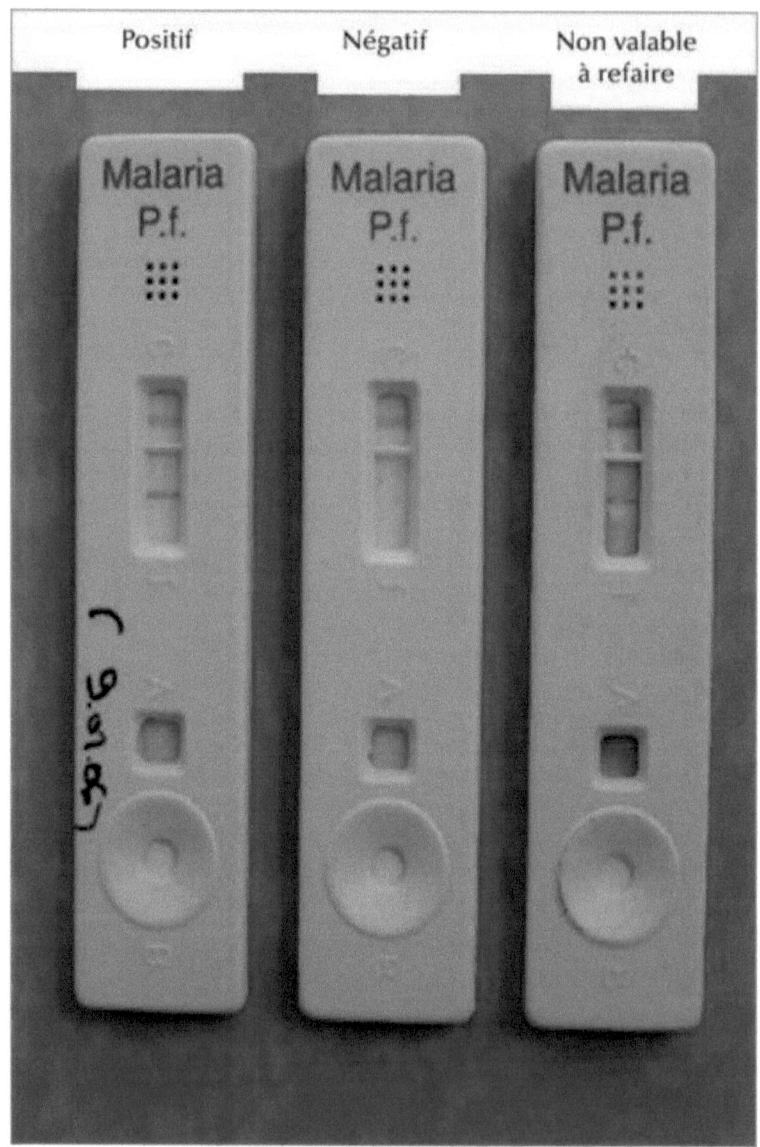

Figure 19: Rësults of the *plasmodium falciparum* RDT.

FACT SHEET

Full name: TRAORE Mahamadou

National^ : Malian

Academic year: 2022-2023

Director of these: Professeur Mahamadou Soumana SISSOKO

Date of defence: 14 November 2023

Email : mahamadoutraore706@gmail.com

Telephone number: 77647584

Title: Profil ëpidëmiologique du paludisme au Centre de San" Communautaire de Мёкт-Sikoro en Commune I du district de Bamako

Sector of interest: Public Health, Epidëmiology, Parasitology

Location of dëpдt: Library of the Facu№ de Pharmacie de Bamako (TAPI I)

Rësumë

Introduction: Malaria is a parasitic disease, a fëbrile and hëmolytic ërythrocytopathy caused by the development and multiplication in humans of Plasmodium mosquitoes. The aim of this study was to assess the management of malaria in the population of Мёкт-Sikoro in 2021.

Methods: This was a cross-sectional ëtude on the ëpidëmiological profile of malaria in Мёкт-Sikoro in commune I of the Bamako district. Notre ëtude, portant sur les registres de consultation et du laboratoire de 2021 et une enquete par interview de 234 personnes tout âge confondu rëalisëe en octobre 2022.

Results: At the end of this study, we observed a malaria incidence rate of 51.5% among CSCOM patients. This frequency varied from one season to another with the maximum number of cases during the rainy season 58.2%. Children aged 6 to 15 suffered more from malaria (57.4%). The most frequent clinical signs ëtait fever %, cëphalëes %, vomiting % and chills %. Simple malaria was the most frequent phënotype 99.5% compared with less than 1% severe malaria. Injectable antimalarial drugs ëwere, however, the most prescribed 73.1%. Antimalarial treatment was correct in 21.2% of cases. The use of insecticide-impregnated mosquito nets was around 66.5%, and 31.1% of pregnant women had received Sulfadoxine-Pyrimethamine. Patients/carers were aware that malaria is transmitted by mosquito bites (77.5%).

Conclusion: Malaria was the most frequent cause of consultation at the Mekin-Sikoro CSCOM. This frequency varied from one season to another, with the highest number of cases in the winter period (July-October), with a high susceptibility among children aged 6-15 years. The most frequent clinical signs were fever, headache, vomiting and chills. Good knowledge of how to prevent malaria

Efforts needed to improve adherence to the national malaria management policy

Key words : Malaria, epidemiology, management

NOTIFICATION FORM

Name & First Name: TRAORE Mahamadou

Nationality : Malian

Academic year : 2022-2023

Director of thesis : Professor Mahamadou Soumana SISSOKO

Date of defense : November 14th,2023

Email : mahamadoutraore706@gmail.com

Phone Number : 77647584

Title: Epidemiological profile of malaria at the Mёкт-Sikoro Community Health Center in Commune I district of Bamako

Sector of interest: Public Health, Epidemiology, Parasitology

Location: Library of the Faculty of Pharmacy

Abstract:

Introduction: Malaria is a parasitic disease, a febrile and hemolyzing erythrocytopathy due to the development and multiplication in humans of hematozoa of the Plasmodium genus. The objective of this work was to evaluate the management of malaria in the population of Mbkin-Sikoro in 2021.

Methods: This was a cross-sectional study on the epidemiological profile of malaria in Mbkin- Sikoro in commune I of the Bamako district. Our study, covering consultation and laboratory registers from 2021 and an interview survey of 234 people of all ages carried out in October 2022.

Results: At the end of this study we observed a malaria frequency of 51.5% among CSCOM patients. This frequency varied from one season to another with the maximum number of cases during winter 58.2%. Children aged 6 to 15 suffered more from malaria 57.4%. The most common clinical signs were fever%, headache%, vomiting% and chills%. Simple malaria was the most frequent phenotype 99.5% compared to less than 1% of severe malaria. However, injectable antimalarials were the most prescribed 73.1%. Antimalarial treatment was correct in 21.2% of cases. The use of insecticide-treated mosquito nets was around 66.5% and 31.1% of pregnant women had received Sulfadoxine-Pyrimethamine. Patients/accompanying people knew that malaria is transmitted by mosquito bites 77.5%.

Conclusion: Malaria was the most frequent cause of consultation at the Mёкт-Sikoro CSCOM. This frequency varied from one season to another with the maximum number of cases in the winter period (July-October) with a high susceptibility of cases in children aged 6-15 years. The most common clinical signs were fever, headache, vomiting and chills. Good knowledge of malaria prevention

Efforts needed to improve adherence to the national malaria management policy

Keywords: Malaria, epidemiology, management

GALEN'S OATH

I swear in the presence of the Masters of this Faculty, the Councillors of the Ordre des Pharmaciens and my dear fellow students.

To honour those who have instructed me in the precepts of my art and to show them my gratitude by remaining faithful to their teaching;

To practise my profession conscientiously in the interests of public health and to comply not only with current legislation but also with the rules of honour, probity and disinterestedness.

Never to forget my responsibility and my duties towards patients and their human dignity. Under no circumstances will I agree to use my knowledge and status to corrupt the wrongdoers and encourage criminal acts.

Respectful and grateful to my teachers, I will give back to their children the education I received from their fathers.

May men think highly of me if I keep my promises.

May I be shamed and despised by my colleagues if I fail to do so.

I swear!

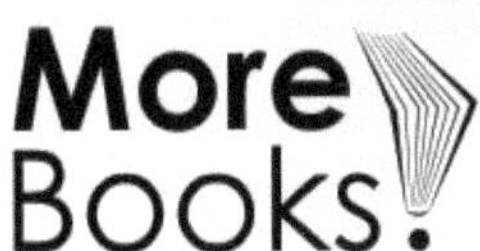

More
Books!

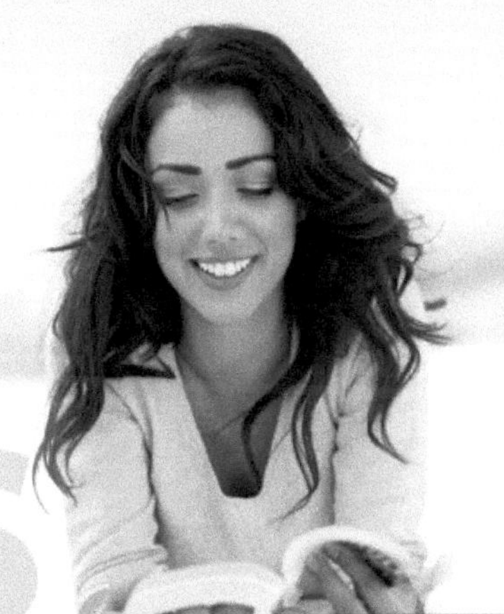

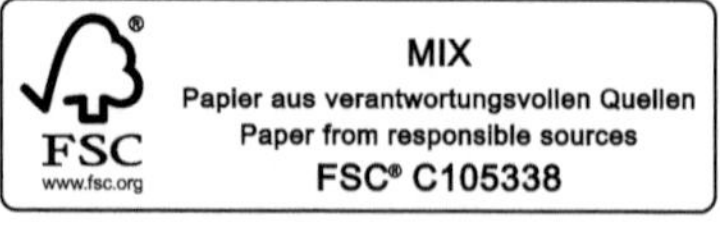

Printed by Books on Demand GmbH, Norderstedt / Germany